THE PSYCHIATRY OF HANDICAPPED CHILDREN AND ADOLESCENTS

THE PSYCHIATRY OF HANDICAPPED CHILDREN AND ADOLESCENTS

MANAGING EMOTIONAL AND BEHAVIORAL PROBLEMS

Joan P. Gerring, M.D.
Department of Developmental Neuropsychiatry
The Kennedy Institute for Handicapped Children
The Johns Hopkins University School of Medicine
Baltimore, Maryland

Lucille Parkinson McCarthy, Ph.D.
Department of Writing and Media
Loyola College
Baltimore, Maryland

A College-Hill Publication
Little, Brown and Company
Boston/Toronto/San Diego

College-Hill Press
A Division of
Little, Brown and Company (Inc.)
34 Beacon Street
Boston, Massachusetts 02108

Library of Congress Cataloging in Publication Data

Main entry under title:

The psychiatry of handicapped children and adolescents.

"A College-Hill publication."
Includes bibliographies and index.
1. Handicapped children. 2. Child psychotherapy.
I. Gerring, Joan P., 1943–   . II. McCarthy, Lucille Parkinson, 1944–
[DNLM: 1. Adolescent Psychiatry. 2. Child Behavior Disorders—
rehabilitation. 3. Child Psychiatry. 4. Education, Special. 5. Handicapped—
psychology. WS 350.6 P9735]
RJ507.H35P77   1988   618.92′89′00880816   87-31048

ISBN 0–316–30844–7

Printed in the United States of America

CONTENTS

PREFACE

Psychiatric problems—emotional and behavioral—are frequently present in handicapped children and adolescents. These problems may accompany the primary handicap, or they may themselves constitute the primary handicap. These emotional and behavioral problems often make evaluation of handicapped youngsters more difficult, and they may, in addition, impede treatment efforts. Because these problems are so common and their consequences so far-reaching, mental health professionals serve as members of comprehensive evaluation and treatment teams in order to identify and treat them. The purpose of this book is to acquaint non-psychiatric specialists with the psychiatric problems of handicapped youth and their treatments. Such knowledge, we believe, will lead to improved communication among specialists, which will, in turn, benefit our students and patients.

Our five contributors have had extensive experience in multidisciplinary work at the Kennedy Institute, Duke University Medical Center, and the Payne Whitney Clinic of the New York Hospital-Cornell Medical Center. In these institutions psychiatric problems are considered an important aspect of the evaluation and treatment of handicapped youngsters.

This book focuses on the ways in which professionals define and treat the emotional and behavioral problems that are presented to them. The first chapter reviews the definition of handicap within the framework of Public Law 94-142 and explains the central role of the public school system in the evaluation and treatment of handicapped youth. It also describes the specialists who provide mental health services and the organization of various kinds of multidisciplinary teams. Chapter 2 describes the psychiatric evaluation and the psychiatric symptoms and disorders which are commonly seen in handicapped youngsters. Chapter 3 focuses on handicapped adolescents, and in Chapter 4 the two most important forms of psychiatric treatment, psychotherapy and drug therapy, are described. Behavioral assessment and treatment of handicapped youth are discussed in Chapter 5, and in Chapters 6 and 7 educational treatments for youngsters with a variety of handicapping conditions are discussed. Specifically, Chapter 6 describes the educational treatment of handicapped youngsters who may also have accompanying psychiatric disorders, and Chapter 7 describes the psychoeducational treatment of children with primary emotional handicaps. Finally, Chapter 8 discusses the family's response and adaptation to their handicapped child.

Many colleagues have helped us in the writing of this book. James Harris, M.D., Director of the Department of Developmental Neuropsychiatry at the Kennedy Institute, has provided continuous and valuable guidance. We wish to thank especially Charles Grob, M.D., Alan Reiss, M.D., Gayle O'Callaghan, Psy.D., and Barbara Buck, M.S.W., for their insightful readings of early drafts of the text. We are also indebted to Yvonne Page and the Kennedy Institute word processing staff for their support, as well as to our editors at College-Hill Press—Marie Linvill and Susan Altman. And, finally, thanks are due to our families for their understanding and encouragement throughout this project.

The impetus for this book developed out of the long friendship and collaboration between Joan Gerring, a child psychiatrist, and Lucille McCarthy, a specialist in the area of medical writing. Dr. Gerring has worked for seven years as a staff psychiatrist and supervisor of psychiatrists-in-training on multidisciplinary teams at The Kennedy Institute for Handicapped Children in Baltimore. Dr. McCarthy teaches writing at Loyola College in Maryland. In addition to medical writing, her research and teaching interests include modern fiction and nonfiction and writing across the curriculum.

FOREWORD

At no time in Western history have children been subjected to so much scrutiny by various professionals. Our modern culture abounds with educators, special educators, speech-language pathologists, psychiatrists, psychologists, rehabilitation specialists, social workers, audiologists, pediatricians, and many more kinds of professionals. They converge on the child in order to provide parents with information and treat and teach their children to help them grow straight. We have infant care books, developmental tomes, and books about adolescence. We espouse adult educational programs that teach parents how to do what our grandparents seem to have done without special instruction. Tradition has been replaced by professionalism—all in the hope that we will raise better products and, as the medical model goes, help and give comfort, but "first of all, not injure."

From the vantage point of parents and professionals, the aims of each professional group are not always realized, partly because we do not understand each other's languages and because our frames of reference differ. Thus, a volume such as this does indeed hold out a unifying hope by creating an *"Esperanto"* to replace the babble of tongues that exists in child care and therapy.

The notion of a team of professionals addressing the problems of the child seems to be a new remedy, but, like all else, the idea is not completely new. During the early years of this century, the Child Guidance Movement in the United States prescribed a division of labor among the members of a team consisting of a social worker, a psychiatrist, and a psychologist. The Child Guidance Movement was, in many ways, an arm of the Mental Hygiene Movement that grew up outside of universities and apart from hospitals, just as the Settlement House idea grew up outside of primary educational institutions and has greater kinship to social welfare and on-site community efforts to influence social development.

Now, during the second half of the century, we again witness attempts at reunification of the many disciplines and professional groups that teach and treat children. Some of these disciplines are more academic, some of them are more practical, but all are clinical, and each directs its attention to the child. The parents' dilemma might be solved by having the team examine the child, with each member applying knowledge from his or her own vantage point. On the other hand, this is not always the case; the primary professional contact frequently is a matter of the referral source's preference and prejudice.

This book goes a long way toward providing information for all professionals who work with children about the frame of reference of their neighbor professions and how we all may work together. What is the alliance that is necessary to help each understand the other? What must we grasp of the other's language to broaden our own vision? In clinical practice it has been all too possible for one professional to criticize the other as "not knowing" or as "incomplete in his or her examination." Parochialism may be bred in the pride that we each take in our own work. On the other hand, the capacity to listen has always been a virtue and should not be strained by the effort necessary to find out what the other fellow has to say. In addition, there have been great advances in special education and language theory, in rehabilitative medicine and behavioral approaches. There have been major changes in traditional dynamic psychotherapy and in the therapeutic nursery for children as well. Each of these advances is explored in this volume by spokespersons who know their work well and practice it too.

In the past, each discipline tended to be practiced in accordance with the old schoolchild chant, "I want to be the Captain or I won't play." However, we have come to a point in history where parents as consumers will no longer tolerate that attitude, nor should they. They take responsibility for the rearing and fixing of their children by making appropriate choices. Obtaining professional help in making such choices does not require that parents relinquish their responsibilities toward their children. Moreover, the professionals who are involved should know that omnipotent fantasies of rescue, adoption, and an attitude of "Only I can save the child" are to be recognized and understood, but *not* acted on.

Dr. Gerring and Dr. McCarthy are to be congratulated for pulling together this compendium of descriptions of how so many people work every day for the betterment of children, and through that effort, for the emergence of better adults too.

Theodore Shapiro, M.D.
Professor of Psychiatry
Cornell University Medical College
Director of Child and Adolescent Psychiatry
Payne Whitney Clinic
New York

CONTRIBUTORS

Elaine Heffner, Ed.D., M.S.W.
Program Supervisor
Nursery School Treatment Center
Payne Whitney Clinic, The New
    York Hospital
New York, New York

Judith M. Levy, M.S.W., L.C.S.W.
Director, Department of Social
    Work
The Kennedy Institute for
    Handicapped Children
Baltimore, Maryland

Lea O'Quinn, M.D.
Assistant Professor of Psychiatry
    and Pediatrics
Duke University Medical Center
Durham, North Carolina

John M. Parrish, Ph.D.
Director of Training and
    Outpatient Services,
    Department of Psychology
The Kennedy Institute for
    Handicapped Children
Assistant Professor, Department of
    Psychiatry
The Johns Hopkins University
    School of Medicine
Baltimore, Maryland

Lois Therres Pommer, Ed.D.
Supervisor of Inpatient and
    Outpatient Evaluation,
School Psychologist II
Special Education Division of
The Kennedy Institute for
    Handicapped Children
Baltimore, Maryland

Thomas M. Reimers, Ph.D.
Postdoctoral Fellow in Behavioral
    Pediatrics
The Johns Hopkins University
    School of Medicine
Baltimore, Maryland

CHAPTER 1

AN OVERVIEW OF HANDICAPPING CONDITIONS AND THE MULTIDISCIPLINARY TEAM APPROACH TO CARE OF HANDICAPPED CHILDREN

Joan P. Gerring and Lucille Parkinson McCarthy

A handicap is a physical or mental impairment that prevents the performance of some necessary and worthwhile activities. Children may have chronic illness or they may have motor, cognitive, psychiatric, or social handicaps. The school system views a handicap as a condition that impairs learning and views the handicapped child as a student who needs special services. Thus, a child who has lost a leg but who still maintains a high level of academic performance will not be seen as handicapped. There are times, however, when differences of opinion arise about what constitutes a handicap or learning impairment. For example, a psychiatrist may view a child as emotionally disturbed, yet the teaching staff may see no behavioral or emotional effect on classroom performance. This child will not be eligible for special services unless the psychiatrist can convince the school staff to accept his or her point of view.

The number of handicapped children and adolescents has increased as the population has increased because a certain percentage of any population will have conditions that hinder development and adjustment. Certain other factors, such as increased longevity, improved techniques of intensive care, and policies of deinstitutionalization also influence the number of handicapped persons in the community.

OVERVIEW OF CARE OF HANDICAPPED CHILDREN

Effects of Medical Advances on Handicapping Conditions

Certain advances in medical technology have lessened the degree of disability associated with handicap. Effective cures have been discovered for many childhood diseases that used to lead to chronic handicaps. Such childhood diseases include poliomyelitis, phenylketonuria, and some types of congenital heart disease. Effective treatment for other diseases has greatly reduced the number of persons who are handicapped from these conditions. For example, medications for childhood tuberculosis, hypothyroidism, and juvenile diabetes have decreased the incidence and severity of subsequent handicaps. In addition, advances have been made in the treatment of infections, such as measles and bacterial pneumonias, for which vaccines and antibiotics have decreased the previously high incidence of death and disability. Cardiac surgery and types of reconstructive surgery have also played important roles in the reduction of childhood death and handicap, as have recently developed effective medications for arthritis, asthma, and epilepsy. The newer area of pediatric nutrition concentrates on disease prevention by careful attention to a good diet in childhood and aims to prevent such chronic handicapping conditions of old age as cardiac disease, stroke, and cancer by promoting healthy eating habits in the young.

Whereas some medical advances have resulted in decreased death rates and fewer subsequent handicaps, other medical advances have resulted in increased survival and a consequent increase in the number of handicapped survivors. Systems of intensive care figure prominently in saving the lives of patients who, in an earlier era, would have died. Neonatal intensive care units now save the lives of very small and very sick infants, who may have poorly functioning digestive, circulatory, or respiratory systems, or other abnormalities, and who formerly would have died. These babies are now supported and strengthened until they can survive without support or until they are able to undergo surgery or other treatments that will eliminate or reduce their abnormalities. After these infants are treated, they may remain in intensive care for long and complicated recovery periods, and they may have handicaps as a result of this early history.

Pediatric medical and surgical intensive care units take care of children who have suffered severe illness or trauma or who are recovering from surgery. Other specialized units include dialysis units where children with poorly functioning or nonfunctioning kidneys may be kept alive for years while they await a kidney transplant. Certain large hospitals have neurological intensive care units where children with severe brain injury or illness are cared for.

Intensive care units have certain features in common. These features include advanced diagnostic techniques such as computed tomography (CT scans) and microblood analyses, specialized mechanical treatments such as respirators and exchange transfusions, and multidisciplinary teams whose members are knowledgeable about the various components of the system. Rapid retrieval of patients, in the case of injury, and rapid diagnosis, in the case of serious illness, are essential to a good outcome. Intensive care is aimed at increased survival, and the outcome may be a complete return to health. Often, however, the outcome is incomplete recovery despite optimal working of the intensive care unit. Infants, children, and adolescents may be left with some amount of handicap. This group of children creates a new population in need of special services.

The precise outcome of most illnesses or injuries is still not possible to predict, although certain helpful guidelines exist. For example, a child who survives 100 days of coma after severe head injury will most likely have at least a moderate degree of chronic handicap. However, a child who survives 2 to 5 days of coma after severe head injury may have mild, moderate, or severe resultant disability or none at all. Such children's outcomes may become apparent only as they go through their periods of recovery. Certain handicaps, such as seizure disorders or emotional disorders, may appear months or even years following the injury. As more is learned about the recovery process following illnesses and injuries, clinicians will better understand the factors that affect patient outcome.

Effects of Deinstitutionalization on Handicapped Children

There has been, since the 1970s, an increase in knowledge and acceptance of handicap. The level of care of handicapped children has also improved and has resulted in increased survival. Previously, many mentally and physically handicapped people were sent to institutions, where they often spent many years, or even their entire lives. In recent years large numbers of physically, mentally, and emotionally handicapped patients have moved from large hospitals or institutions back into community living settings and meaningful activities. This deinstitutionalization movement is a response both to the many abuses that existed in the former system and to a raised public concern for the rights of all people. Another impetus for deinstitutionalization of the emotionally handicapped was the optimistic belief that the use of major tranquilizers would lead to a decrease in these people's needs for services. Institutional life often resulted in physical and mental deterioriation, whereas community life would allow the handicapped to mingle with the nonhandicapped and to maintain the highest possible level of functioning. For example, it was rare for an autistic child with normal intellectual potential to maintain a high intelligence quotient (IQ) after several years of institutional care. By contrast, autistic adolescents with normal intellectual potential are now commonly seen in specialized day schools in the community.

The increased visibility of handicapped people in the community has contributed to increased awareness of the handicapped, of who they are and of what their needs are. They are now viewed as members of families and community groups. Deinstitutionalization also presents problems, however. Families who are raising a handicapped child in the home often are unable to deal with all of the aspects of care without assistance. Sometimes many services are necessary for a single child, and the ancillary services formerly available under one roof in an institution may be widely scattered or unavailable to an individual family.

As a minority population, handicapped persons have profited from the increased attention being paid to their potentials and the needs of all minorities. The legal movement for racial equality in the schools in the 1950s and 1960s gave impetus to the creation of a comprehensive educational program for the handicapped in the 1970s. Handicapped people have received a great deal of support from alliances with other minorities and have shared productive strategies with these groups.

Support Organizations for Handicapped Persons

To obtain and coordinate services for children with various handicaps in the community, parents and involved professionals have joined together to form organizations to assist them. These organizations are support-giving and task-oriented. They begin by surveying the needs of their particular population and the possible service resources that exist in the community, focusing both on adapting existing resources and creating new ones. These organizations also work to educate the public, and some are large enough to support considerable research efforts.

These organizations for handicapped persons have worked effectively through the legislative and judicial systems to address specific needs. Some large organizations have lobbyists and lawyers who work on issues of special interest to their clients. Their members also elicit support from legislators and serve as advocates in lawsuits to obtain better services for their particular groups. Often an organization seeking to influence legislation will ally itself with other interested organizations to strengthen its position. Over the years, these organizations have achieved many advances for their clients.

Results of Passage of Public Law 94-142 (PL 94-142)

Passage in 1975 of Public Law 94-142, the Education for All Handicapped Children Act, resulted in the organization of services for the handicapped that exist today. This law redefined education for handicapped children to include rehabilitation and other related services. The antecedents for this landmark legislation come from the increased efforts beginning in the 1950s to ensure educational equality for all minority groups. The *Brown vs. Board of Education* decision in 1954 defined equal education for all students as a constitutional right (Wright, 1982). Federal legislation in the 1960s gave scholarship aid to teachers of handicapped children (Community Mental Health and Retardation Act, 1963), directed funds to the education of economically disadvantaged youth (Elementary and Secondary Education Act, 1965), created the Bureau of Education for the Handicapped (Education of the Handicapped Act, 1966), and supported grants and model programs in study areas of specific handicaps and early childhood development.

In 1971, a Pennsylvania court ruled that the school system had to provide education to retarded children, who had until then been deemed uneducable. The court further decided that the evaluation and placement of these handicapped students must involve due process to protect the rights of the child and his or her family. This court decision, referred to as the Pennsylvania Association of Retarded Citizens' decision, was made as the United States Congress began the 4 years of study that resulted in passage of the Education for All Handicapped Children Act in 1975.

PL 94-142 provided federal support for comprehensive and appropriate education of handicapped children from 3 to 21 years of age with due process provided to the parents. States were required to develop plans to be carried out at the state and local levels that fulfilled the requirements of the federal law (Martin, 1985; Wright, 1982).

The provision and coordination of these educational-rehabilitation services has become the responsibility of the public school system. *The definition of educational services has been extended to include services that will enable the handicapped person to live a productive life in his or her community.* These related educational services include some health care, physical and occupational therapies, and mental health counseling. As a result of this global involvement of the school system in the lives of many handicapped children, current educational procedures and policies are extremely relevant to the subject of this book: the emotional and behavioral problems of handicapped youngsters.

Agencies outside the school provide important treatments and other services, and their role in educating and rehabilitating the handicapped is extremely important. These agencies often work in close cooperation with the schools, sometimes with contractual arrangements. State departments of special education and the local educational associations have gained a primary role in obtaining and coordinating services, however.

Early Intervention in Educating Handicapped Children

The needs of handicapped children are being addressed at a younger age. PL 94-142 extended educational services to include 3-year-old children, and thus many states have created programs to serve handicapped children from ages 3 to 5 years old. PL 99-457, the Education of the Handicapped Amendments of 1986, further extended federal involvement in early childhood education to include the special needs of handicapped infants and toddlers from birth through 2 years of age. Early intervention programs identify disadvantaged young children and young children who are at high risk for the development of handicaps. These children are evaluated and areas of present or potential deficit receive special attention from trained personnel. Although many handicapped children are now in early intervention programs, only those early intervention programs with blind, deaf, and language disordered children have actually proved to be beneficial (Fraiberg and Fraiberg, 1979; Horton, 1974). The effects of early intervention in all other handicaps have not yet been established scientifically (Martin, 1985).

When a potential handicap has been identified and evaluated, therapy is then designed to focus on the individual needs of the child. Parents may be taught to administer the therapy and to stimulate their child with tasks that permit success. A review of early intervention studies points to the benefit of these programs in improved family functioning (Simeonsson, Cooper, and Scheiner, 1982). Such programs involve parents in a number of ways. Parents are educated about their child's disability, and mental health workers help them develop healthy coping skills while discouraging maladaptive activities. Because mothers of very dependent handicapped children experience more stress than do mothers with children who need less care (Breslau, Staruch, and Mortimer, 1982), workers help parents construct schedules to ease the workload with these children. Such interventions, it is hoped, will lead to improved mother-child interactions.

Child Find is a component of many special education programs that identify potentially handicapped children. In the state of Maryland, for example, Child Find identifies children from birth through 5 years of age. After referral by parent or professional, pertinent background material is collected, and the child is evaluated for the presence of handicaps that may interfere with his or her learning. If a handicap is identified, Child Find arranges placement within the special education system, or, if necessary, arranges for the provision of services with outside agencies. Programs for children younger than 3 years old emphasize parental involvement along with appropriate services. At age 3 years, many of the children are placed in half-day, early-childhood intervention classes that often provide ancillary services, such as physical and occupational therapy and speech and language services. Some children may continue in a Child Find kindergarten program prior to placement in a regular or special education first grade.

FACTORS AFFECTING A CHILD'S ADJUSTMENT TO A HANDICAP

Children and adolescents may have a variety of handicapping conditions, and a particular child may have just one handicap or several. Before exploring specific handicapping conditions, however, consideration will be given to some general factors that may affect youngsters' emotional and psychological adjustments to their handicaps.

Onset of Handicap

The onset of a handicap may have relevance to the emotional life of the handicapped person. Some handicaps are present at birth, and other handicaps have their onset after birth. When a handicap is present from birth, the child's personality develops and adjusts in relation to the handicap. He or she incorporates the handicap into his self-image and personality, and hopes for the future are all related to the handicap that the child has always possessed. He or she may not be ashamed or shy, even if the handicap is a physical disfigurement.

When the onset of handicap is gradual, the child has time to adjust slowly to it. His or her reaction will depend on the severity of impairment and on his or her personality structure. A child who has reacted to stressful situations in the past with anger will likely respond to the stress of illness with anger. Other children may respond with denial, deterioration of school performance, or aggressive behavior.

In addition to congenital and gradual onset of handicaps, handicaps may be of sudden onset. This type may occur in a previously unimpaired child. A severe accident—for example, a paralyzing spinal cord injury—may cause great psychological stress, for which the child is likely to be unprepared. A formerly independent child with normal activity and behavior is now helpless and totally dependent.

The sudden onset of handicap in a child creates an acute family crisis. All of the family's resources must be mobilized during the period of intensive care. When their child's survival is ensured, the family reacts and adjusts over a period of years to the persistence of the handicap, mourning the loss of the child who was once unimpaired and without problems. Just as children react to noncongenital handicaps according to previous patterns of response, families also react to a newly handicapped child according to their previous patterns of response. Parents may be able to adapt easily to the new circumstances, or they may have a variety of adjustment problems. Family response and adjustment are explored further in Chapter 8.

Visibility of Handicap

Another factor that may affect the youngster's emotional and psychological adjustment to a handicap is how apparent the handicap is. A facial or hand disfigurement is visible and apparent, whereas a severe congenital heart ailment or a developmental reading disability may be inapparent to an observer. A person may have a physical abnormality that may be major or minor, such as a chest deformity, but it is not apparent because it is usually covered by clothing. Epilepsy is a condition in which handicap may be apparent only when the person is having a seizure. Any of these handicaps may have psychological concomitants in the patient and may engender psychological reactions in the families. The psychological influence of the handicap may reflect less the actual handicap than it does the ways in which the patient and family come to view it. The psychological meaning of even a minor, inapparent abnormality may be exaggerated if it is connected to a powerful, aggressive fantasy developed by the patient (Niederland, 1980). In the Isle of Wight study, psychiatric disorder appeared to be no more common in patients with visible handicaps than in patients with handicaps that were not visible (Graham and Rutter, 1968).

Effects of Handicap on Mobility

Certain handicaps restrict movement or immobilize the patient, and this may also affect children's adjustments to their handicaps. An infant may be immobilized in a cast because of clubfoot or hip dislocation, or a young child with cerebral palsy may need metal braces to assist in ambulation. The movements of a blind toddler must be supervised carefully, and a teenager with muscular dystrophy has severe muscle weakness and is no longer able to walk. A young girl with a spinal cord injury after trauma is confined to her wheelchair. Restriction of movement influences psychological functioning according to the developmental stage of the child and the duration of the immobility. An immobilized toddler will not have the same opportunity to explore his or her surroundings as the child who is free to run. And he or she might not be able to demonstrate feelings of aggression and affection as easily. If the immobilization is brief, it may have little subsequent influence on the child's functioning. By contrast, permanent confinement will likely lead to a more lasting influence on personality formation. Restriction of movement for an older child often results in lessened opportunity for social interactions, and an impaired ability to walk usually lengthens the time a teenager is dependent on the family. If restriction of movement is accompanied by deficiencies in the functional skills of toileting, dressing, and eating, the time of dependency may be even longer.

HANDICAPS THAT IMPAIR LEARNING

Handicaps that impair learning are emphasized in this book. Although all states subscribe to PL 94-142, individual state by-laws differ somewhat in their definitions of handicapping conditions and the categories of services they provide. Table 1–1 lists the most important groups of conditions that receive educational attention. Chapters 6 and 7 focus specifically on the educational management of children with learning disabilities, orthopedic impairments, mental retardation, and pervasive developmental disorders. In this chapter all the groups of handicapping conditions are defined and discussed briefly. Chapter 2 describes the psychiatric conditions that may accompany them.

Mental Retardation

Mental retardation refers to significantly below average intellectual functioning along with deficits in adaptive behavior. This combination is first manifested during a child's development, with onset before 18 years of age (American Association on Mental Deficiency, 1983). The level of intellectual functioning is assessed by standardized intelligence tests, and PL 94-142 stipulates that tests be chosen to encourage optimal performance in the child. Commonly used instruments include the Wechsler Intelligence Scale for Children–Revised (WISC-R), the

TABLE 1–1.
Conditions that Impair Learning

Mental retardation	Emotional disturbances
Learning disabilities	Physical illnesses and abnormalities
Language disabilities	Other neurological handicaps
Speech disorders	Orthopedic disorders
Visual impairments	Multiple handicaps
Hearing impairments	Pregnancy

Stanford-Binet Intelligence Scale, and the Cattell Infant Intelligence Scale.

Adaptive functioning is also assessed by standardized scales such as the Vineland Adaptive Behavior Scales and the American Association on Mental Deficiency (AAMD) Adaptive Behavior Scales. Adaptive scales should measure functioning in specific areas, including self-help skills, communication skills, number and time use, and socialization. Emotional and motivational behavior are also measured on these scales. Because skills measured on intelligence tests contribute to total adaptation, the intelligence quotient correlates with the level of adaptive behavior. Discrepancies can occur between IQ and the level of adaptive functioning, however (American Association on Mental Deficiency, 1983). For example, a child may appear to be functioning at a higher intellectual level because he or she has many positive behaviors that enhance a more limited intellectual response. Alternatively, sometimes a child's behavioral repertoire is so limited or so maladaptive that his or her general level of intellectual functioning seems to be lower than it has been measured.

There are four commonly accepted levels of retardation, each level measured by both intellectual and adaptive standards. These levels are mild, moderate, severe, and profound and are measured by standardized, individual tests. An error of measurement of 3 to 4 points gives every stated IQ a range of 6 to 8 IQ points. For example, an IQ of 55 represents an IQ zone from 51–52 to 58–59. The level of adaptive behavior, measured by a behavioral scale or by clinical evaluation, is taken into consideration in making the determination of retardation level. An IQ level below 70 in verbal and performance tests and in adaptive behavior indicates that the child is retarded. Children or adolescents who have IQs below 70 experience difficulties in academic or adaptive functioning and will need special education and other special services. It is estimated that 2.7 to 3 percent of the population have IQs below 70 (Reid, 1980). In 1970, 2,800,000 youths of ages less than 1 to 21 years were estimated to be mentally retarded (Kakalik et al., 1973).

Mild Retardation

A mildly retarded child or adolescent has an IQ range from 50–55 to approximately 70. About 90 percent of retarded people fall within this range of IQ. Most mildly retarded children have family histories of retardation with members showing varying levels of retardation. These children generally grow normally and have unremarkable appearance. They live at home and are not often institutionalized. Mildly retarded people progress by their late teens to about the sixth grade level of academic functioning. The mildly retarded marry, but their reproductive rate is less than that of people with normal intelligence. As adults, they can attain the vocational and social skills necessary for semi-skilled employment. However, guidance may be needed in handling finances or in dealing with complicated matters such as health care or legal problems.

Moderate, Severe, and Profound Retardation

Moderately, severely, and profoundly retarded groups, as defined by the American Association on Mental Deficiency (1973), share characteristics not present in the mildly retarded, and so it has become common to speak of children and adolescents with IQs below 50 as severely retarded. The prevalence rate of severe mental retardation is about 4 per 1,000 persons (Abramowicz and Richardson, 1975). People with Down syndrome constitute about one-third of this group. Severely retarded children have high mortality rates within the first 5 years of life. Their growth and head circumference are often abnormal, and they have a high incidence of nervous system abnormalities, such as cerebral palsy and seizures. Frequently they are sterile. More boys than girls are severely retarded. Most severely retarded children are single cases in families, but if another family member is retarded, the level of retardation will be similar. Developmental retardation usually appears early in these severely impaired children. Associated physical and neurological problems also bring these children to early medical attention.

MODERATE RETARDATION. The AAMD's moderately retarded group has an IQ range of 35–40 to 50–55. Most patients with Down syndrome fall within this IQ level. The moderately retarded can learn to talk or communicate and may attain the second grade academic level by their late teenage years. Their performance of activities of daily living and their social interaction abilities may be good. Moderately retarded individuals may receive vocational training in preparation for unskilled or semi-skilled employment in sheltered workshops. Most moderately retarded children live at home and attend special education facilities in the community.

SEVERE RETARDATION. Severe retardation in the AAMD classification includes the IQ range from 20–25 to 35–40. These children may be trained in simple feeding and dressing skills and hygiene. Simple speech may develop, and simple, routine shopping and household tasks may be performed with supervision, but vocational training usually is not successful. Severely retarded children are cared for in their homes and in institutions.

PROFOUND RETARDATION. Profoundly retarded individuals in the AAMD classification are in the IQ range below 20 to 25. These children and adolescents need constant care and supervision, although they may assist in their self-care to a limited degree. Simple speech may or may not develop by the teenage years. If speech does not develop, these children may use gestures to communicate their needs.

Learning Disabilities

Learning disabilities refer to specific deficits in academic performance in children who are average or near average in intelligence. By 1985 the learning disabled population represented 4 percent of the total school population (Martin, 1985). The definition of learning disability varies among the states according to how far behind a child must be in specified academic areas. In Maryland, a child must be 2 years or more behind in a subject to be classified as learning disabled. To qualify for special education, the learning disability cannot be the result of cultural or environmental factors nor because of the presence of another handicap. This distinction is often difficult to make, as multiple factors may be present in a child and may contribute to the appearance and persistence of a learning disability. For example, a child from a disorganized, culturally deprived family may first come to attention because of long-standing reading backwardness first noted after the death of a family member. An innate reading deficit may be only a contributing factor to reading problems in such a child.

Language Disorders

Expressive and receptive language deficits may impede academic progress. Expressive language ability is the ability to communicate using spoken or written words. Receptive language ability refers to the degree of comprehension of spoken or written words. It is estimated that up to 5 percent of children have deficient acquisition of oral or written language, or both (Resnick, Allen, and Rapin, 1984). A child who is not using words by age 18 months or is not using phrases to communicate by age 24 months should be referred for language evaluation. Children demonstrating language impairment in preschool or in elementary school are referred to speech-language pathologists for evaluation and treatment planning. A neuropsychologist, if one is available, can help to define a profile of cognitive and neurodevelopmental skills that will help the multidisciplinary team to construct an educational program for the language impaired child. Dysphasias, or developmental language disorders, must be distinguished from language impairments attributable to hearing loss, mental retardation, or emotional disorders. The aim of treatment is to help the child develop an effective means of communicating, using speech or some other method.

Children with language deficits have a high frequency of psychiatric disorders, and these disorders do not seem to cluster in any particular category (Gualtieri, Koriath, VanBourgondien, and Saleeby, 1983). Surveys have found psychiatric symptoms in from 44 to 84 percent of language impaired children. The frequency of developmental language disorders is also high in child psychiatry inpatients.

Speech Disorders

Speech disorders have multiple causes, including mental retardation, developmental or acquired language disabilities, deafness, and defects of anatomy, such as cleft palate or absent larynx. Speech disorders may accompany language disorders or may occur as a solitary handicap. Dysarthria is a type of speech disorder resulting from dysfunction of the muscles that control speech. Both genetic and environmental factors play important roles in the onset and persistence of stuttering, another important speech disorder. A child of 18 months who is not speaking or who has unintelligible speech should be referred to a developmental pediatrician for evaluation. The aim of treatment for children with speech disorders is to help them communicate by use of speech or an alternative form of communication. The more severe the speech or language impairment, the more important the need for a comprehensive program that includes parental involvement and the opportunity for counseling.

Visual Impairment

A spectrum of visual handicaps exists. Legal blindness is defined as a distant visual acuity of 20–200 or less in the better eye with correction. It is also defined as a field of vision that subtends an angle of 20 degrees or less. The term legal blindness gives some indication of the need for services but does not give much information about functional capability. Most visually handicapped children are partially sighted and are able to use printed material to learn. Such youths number 1 in 500 school-aged children according to estimates by the National Society for the Prevention of Blindness. More severely affected children are unable to read printed material and must be prepared to use braille and to develop special listening and tactile skills.

Motor and social development is often delayed in children with visual impairment. These children sit, crawl, and walk at later ages than other children, and decreased eye contact and smiling may interfere with the development of the mother-child relationship. A milestone in the development of personality that may be delayed in the visually impaired child is the knowledge that the mother and other objects exist even when they are not present.

Children with visual impairment are evaluated for school placement using specifically designed tests. In planning a child's educational program, careful attention is paid to psychological factors, such as motivation, self-esteem, and interpersonal relatedness. Prior to passage of PL 94-142, most children with severe visual handicaps attended residential schools. Now integrated programs within the public school system exist for blind children who do not have multiple handicaps and who have fairly good social adjustment. These programs enable visually handicapped children to live at home and to attend a combination of regular and resource classes. In addition, there still are segregated day and residential schools that offer blind children comprehensive academic programs and small classes through the secondary level. In such schools, orientation and mobility training are emphasized (Nelson, 1984).

Hearing Impairment

The spectrum of sensorineural hearing impairment ranges from mild to profound and may affect the development of speech and language. Measured as decibels (dB) of sound loss, mild hearing loss begins at about 25 dB HL (decibels hearing level) and may delay speaking and cause subsequent academic problems. Severe bilateral sensorineural loss begins at about 65 dB and is suffered by about 1 in 1000 people. If the loss is mild, the child can learn language by auditory amplification and other types of intervention. At severe levels of loss (about 75 dB or greater), alternative communication methods, such as signing, may be necessary. Generally the less severe the loss, the older the child is before the loss is detected. Research indicates that early intervention with severe and profound hearing losses has a pronounced positive effect on expressive language development compared with intervention after the age of 3 years (Brannon and Murray, 1966; Matkin, 1984). Neonatal screening programs have not been very successful in detecting newborns with mild or moderate degrees of hearing impairment. It remains for the parents and the pediatrician to suspect hearing impairment in the preschool child. Referral to hearing specialists should be made when there is a deficiency in age-appropriate number and clarity of words and phrases produced and responded to.

Emotional Disturbance

An emotional disorder may be a child's only handicapping condition. Emotional disorders, which include a wide range of psychiatric and behavioral problems, affected an estimated 1,500,000 youths in 1970 (Kakalik et al., 1973). These disorders range from disruptive or aggressive behavior to mood disorders of depression, fearfulness, and anxiety. Autism and other disturbances of social, language, and cognitive development are also types of emotional disorders. To qualify for a special education placement for an emotional handicap, a child must have a disorder of sufficient severity to interfere with his or her academic progress. The disorders may be short-term, or they may have a more chronic course.

The severity of the emotional disturbance and its interference with academic progress is judged by the referring school system and the evaluating psychiatrist or psychologist. Teachers identify the behaviors and emotional problems that impair learning in the classroom and judge their severity by the resulting academic impairment or disruption. The school report assists the psychiatrist or psychologist in evaluating the student. He or she then translates psychiatric terms into language that the school system can use in making a suitable educational plan. For example, in addition to reporting that a child has a reactive depression, the psychiatrist must explain why the child is seriously emotionally disturbed and then suggest the type of school program that will alleviate the consequent learning impairment. As the psychiatrist and the educator view the child from their own professional perspectives, different impressions are certain to emerge. The multidisciplinary meeting is an excellent setting in which to gain additional input and work toward a consensus about proper management. If team discussion is not feasible, a conversation between the teacher and the psychiatrist or psychologist usually helps to define a common impression and a suitable treatment plan.

Physical Illnesses and Abnormalities

The educator and the physician participate in the evaluation and educational planning for children with chronic illnesses. The type of illness, its severity, and its duration all figure in the educational and medical evaluation of the student. Learning limitations such as decreased strength, energy, or alertness are determined, and a program is constructed to focus on the child's particular needs. Chronic illnesses that may adversely affect educational performance include asthma, heart disease, arthritis, and kidney disease.

In Baltimore, Maryland, the Home and Hospital Services administer the educational programs for children with chronic illnesses or disabilities. Teachers in this program are trained both to recognize psychiatric problems that interfere with learning and to refer affected students for evaluation. Home and Hospital Services, part of the Division of Public Services in Special Education, conducts four educational programs. Home Teaching and Tele-Teaching are two programs of instruction that take place in the student's home. In addition, nine hospital schools have been established that provide extended programs for many school-aged children. A fourth program, the Chronic Health Impaired Program, provides educational and related services to children who have chronic illnesses and thus must attend school sporadically (The Upton School, 1984). A counseling service for students and their families is an important part of this program.

Other Neurological Handicaps

Neurological handicaps may be temporary, lasting only weeks or months, as in an episode of meningitis. Alternatively, such handicaps may be permanent, as in paralysis resulting from a fall. These disabilities may or may not affect the brain and its function. Traumatic head injury and meningitis are neurological disorders that do affect brain function, whereas paralysis of the lower extremities has no such effect. Epileptic children often have learning and emotional problems. These problems may accompany the epilepsy or may be a reaction to the illness or its drug treatment.

Educational treatment of a child with a neurological handicap varies according to the nature of the condition and the type and degree of learning impairment that results from the particular disability. A child recovering from severe traumatic brain injury may have long-lasting cognitive, motor, and psychiatric deficits and may need a comprehensive school program providing many therapeutic services. A child with lesser brain injury may use home teaching or a transitional school program before returning to a regular classroom. A child recovering from meningitis may attend a hospital school and then receive home teaching before returning to his or her former classroom (if there are no resultant deficits) or being placed in a special education program (if there are persistent deficits). A child who is paralyzed after a fall may receive home and hospital teaching, followed by return to his or her regular class.

Cerebral palsy is a neurological handicap that affects a child's movement and coordination. The estimated incidence of this handicap is 1 to 2 cases per 1000 live births (Stanley, 1982). An infant may or may not have symptoms suggestive of cerebral palsy prior to 1 year of age. The abnormal tone and reflexes characteristic of the disorder tend to appear at the end of the first year and to evolve as the child matures. The clinical picture varies according to the type of cerebral palsy that develops, but the degree of a child's handicap is complete by about 3 years of age, and there is no further progression.

A number of theories of causation have been entertained, but the cause of most cases of cerebral palsy is still unknown. Risk factors, including mental retardation of the mother, prematurity, and a malformation of the baby observed before or at birth, alert the family and the pediatrician to carefully follow the baby's motor development (Nelson and Ellenberg, 1986). Parents may notice that one hand makes a persistent fist, there is a delay in achieving certain developmental milestones, or there is prolonged drooling as the first indication of motor abnormality. Several types of cerebral palsy occur, each with different neurological and motor abnormalities. Spastic cerebral palsy, which includes hemiplegia (stiff and weak, contracted muscles of both extremities on the same side) and diplegia (stiff and weak, contracted muscles with greater involvement of the lower than the upper limbs) is the most common type.

Early intervention plays an important role in the educational planning for the child with cerebral palsy. Referred children are assessed for the presence of multiple handicaps and then are placed in intervention programs that include education for the child and support to help the families accept and understand their child's handicap and to adapt to his or her chronic care needs. There is, however, no evidence that these programs affect the motor aspects of the child's handicap significantly. When the child reaches school age, his or her level of handicap will be reassessed, and the child will then enter a special education or a regular school program.

Orthopedic Disorders

Orthopedic disorders are temporary or permanent disorders of the skeletal system that result in impaired movement. Most childhood and adolescent fractures are uncomplicated, with a cast being placed and rapid return to the classroom. Children with complicated fractures may need a period of hospitalization followed by home teaching. Skeletal diseases, such as severe scoliosis or malignancy, may need inpatient treatment and involve prolonged convalescence. Children with chronic inherited diseases that affect the skeleton, such as the mucopolysaccharidoses and osteogenesis imperfecta, may need special school programs to help them achieve and maintain their academic potential.

Multiple Handicaps

A child who has more than one handicap is said to be multiply handicapped. Certain handicapping conditions are frequently seen together. These include deafness and blindness, retardation and emotional disorders, and language disorders and learning disabilities. Cerebral palsy is a neurological handicap that also has a number of associated handicaps (see Table 1-3). The greater the number and severity of handicaps, the greater the need for multiple services and for coordination of services. Family adjustment tends to be more difficult when multiple handicaps are present because of the perception of greater damage and because of the increased difficulty of care. Moreover, a multiply handicapped child is more vulnerable to the development of psychological problems than is a child with a single handicap. The ability to cope and to adapt to circumstances of daily life is often compromised by the presence of multiple deficits.

Pregnancy

Because learning may be interrupted or impaired during pregnancy, it is viewed by Texas state law as a handicapping condition. Pregnancy is a major psychosocial problem for adolescents and extends far beyond the birth of the child. Pregnancy is an important reason why teenagers in the United States fail to finish high school, and many of these teenaged parents will remain undereducated and underskilled. Their babies have a higher incidence of prematurity, low birth weight, and subsequent learning and behavioral problems. Special education programs provide the option of regular or special classrooms for pregnant teenagers, where classes on parenting and infant nutrition may be provided. The goal of these educational programs is reintegration of the teenager into academic or vocational high school programs.

TABLE 1–2.
Handicaps Associated with Cerebral Palsy

Mental retardation	Hearing impairment
Learning disabilities	Neurological handicaps—
Language disabilities	epilepsy, central sensory impairment
Speech handicaps—dysarthria	Orthopedic disorders—
Visual impairment	scoliosis, subluxation of the hip

MENTAL HEALTH COUNSELING FOR
HANDICAPPED CHILDREN

Education-Related Services

PL 94-142 provides for related services to enable a handicapped student to profit from an education. Counseling of the student is one of these services. Counseling is also provided for parents to help them understand and provide for their child's educational needs. Psychiatric problems may occur in a handicapped child in one of three ways: (1) they may not be present when the handicapped student first enters special education but may appear later; (2) the psychiatric problems may already be present when the handicapped student enters special education; (3) a psychiatric problem may be the main reason why special education services are needed. Three examples will illustrate.

In the first example, the child's psychiatric problem *develops after he or she has entered special education.* A moderately retarded 8-year-old boy with cerebral palsy, for example, develops aggressive behavior in the classroom although there was no prior history of aggression. This behavior impedes his progress and disrupts the classroom. The educational staff, with the consultation of a psychiatrist or psychologist, evaluates the reasons for the aggression and devises a plan to decrease or eliminate the behavior. If counseling is recommended to assist school functioning, the school system provides the service. The school designates one of its own mental health personnel or contracts outside for the service. This student's behavior would be viewed as a temporary disruption in his progress.

In the second example, the child *enters special education with a psychiatric problem in addition to his primary handicap.* A moderately retarded 8-year-old boy with cerebral palsy, for example, comes to evaluation with a 3-year history of aggressive behavior. His behavior is a major consideration in the initial special education evaluation and placement. The teacher and the mental health consultant (the psychiatrist or psychologist) work together to investigate the sources and nature of the child's aggression and to tailor a treatment program that takes the retardation, the physical handicap, and the aggressive behavior into consideration. The focus of the program will be to ensure that educational progress is made by both the child and his classmates. To treat and control this 8-year-old boy's aggression, his program might take place in a small, highly structured class and include the use of a behavioral management protocol.

In the third example, the child *comes for special education evaluation with severe aggressive behavior as his or her only handicap.* The child is an

8-year-old boy, for example. His intelligence is in the normal range and he has no physical impairment, but he is unable to function in a regular classroom. This child's educational plan will reflect his primary emotional handicap. The psychiatrist, psychologist, and special educator will construct a curriculum that provides age-appropriate school work with continual attention paid to the emotional needs of the student. Education of such a child takes place in a special setting and is carried out by staff members trained to work with patients who are emotionally disturbed.

The management of the psychiatric problem is different in each of the three situations just described and depends on the intensity of the problem, its duration, and the coexistence of other handicaps.

It is important for professionals to be aware of the psychiatric problems of handicapped persons because many handicapped children and adolescents have behavioral or emotional problems at one time or another. Professionals working with handicapped youngsters are expected to recognize these problems and to help formulate effective treatments.

Most persons working with handicapped people, however, have not been trained to recognize and to deal effectively with emotional and behavioral problems in their clients. Members of the staff—for example, the teacher, the speech pathologist, the physical therapist, or the bus driver—may notice that a child's behavior is negative or extreme or strange. The behavior may be new to the child, or it may be one that he or she has had for a long time. In any case, the staff member is concerned about the negative effect of the behavior on the child's relationship with staff and with other children. In addition, the staff member's job becomes more difficult as a result of the child's behavior problem. For example, in class or in therapy, work with that child is less effective, and less is accomplished during a session. The child is too active or too sad or too distracted to profit from what is being taught, and this behavior may disrupt the work of the other children. Alternatively, if the child is on a school bus and begins to fight with a classmate, his or her behavior jeopardizes the safety of everyone on the bus. These behaviors upset the staff because their task becomes more difficult, and consequently they may lose the gratification that they experience when their job is done well. Staff members may get discouraged and question their own abilities. At times they may devote many extra hours to a difficult student and become involved with the family in the hope that this personal contact will result in improvement. In some cases, however, no amount of effort will improve the situation; the behavior will not change, and it may even become worse. Because these situations arise frequently, it is important that all persons who care for handicapped children be able to recognize a range of psychiatric problems in their clients and be able to work with other staff members to define the problem and formulate a treatment plan.

When a child's behavioral or emotional problem is brought up for discussion in a staff meeting, people working with the child describe the behavior or change in behavior as it affects them. This description is the first step in treatment. Psychiatrists and psychologists can assist in this process by asking questions and providing terminology, but the basic task of observing and describing the child's problem behavior belongs to the staff members who work with the child.

Incidence of Psychiatric Disorders in Handicapped Children

Psychiatric disorders are more common in the handicapped than in the normal population. Child psychiatrists describe a high incidence of behavioral and emotional problems in retarded populations. Chess followed 52 mentally retarded children for a period of up to 6 years. These middle class children were living at home and ranged in age from 5 to 12 years at the beginning of the study. All of the children were raised in a positive environment and had parents dedicated to their well-being. The children's IQs ranged from 50 to 75. At the initial evaluation, 31 of 52 children (60 percent) fulfilled criteria for behavioral disorder. At the 3 year follow-up, 28 of 48 children (58 percent) fulfilled these criteria. At the 6-year follow-up, 18 of 44 children (41 percent) evidenced behavioral disorder (Chess and Hassibi, 1970).

Other studies also describe a high incidence of behavioral and emotional problems in retarded populations. Menolascino evaluated 616 children 8 years of age and younger who were referred to an outpatient evaluation unit with a clinical suspicion of mental retardation. A multidisciplinary clinical staff described 191 of the 616 children (31 percent) as having prominent psychiatric problems at the time of the evaluation (Menolascino, 1971). In a third study, Szymanski (1977) evaluated 132 consecutive patients referred to an evaluation clinic because of developmental delay. One hundred and six of these 132 patients were retarded. Of the retarded group, 57 children (54 percent) had psychiatric problems that needed attention. Twenty-five of these children had previously been seen in the clinic primarily for evaluation of severe psychiatric problems. These studies all indicate that retarded people are far more likely than their normal counterparts to suffer from emotional and behavioral problems.

The Isle of Wight survey performed in England provides the best information about the incidence of psychiatric problems in children with other types of handicaps (Graham and Rutter, 1968). The survey included 11,865 Isle of Wight school children, aged 5 through 14 years, with a variety of handicapping conditions. Mentally retarded children

were *not* included in the study, however, and multiple screening procedures were used to identify children with other selected handicaps.
One group included children with epilepsy, cerebral palsy, and other
brain conditions. These children and their parents were interviewed
and tested by specialists that included psychiatrists, psychologists, and
physicians with neurological training, and reports were obtained from
schools, hospitals, and other agencies. Comparison groups were composed of (1) children from the general population and (2) children with
chronic physical handicaps not involving the nervous system.

The rate of psychiatric problems among children from the general
population was 6.8 percent. The rate of psychiatric problems among
the children with chronic physical handicaps not involving the brain
was almost twice that (11.5 percent). And the rate of psychiatric problems in the epileptic group was five times that of the general population (34.3 percent). Furthermore, low IQ and reading retardation were
strongly associated with psychiatric disorders in both the general
population and the epileptic children. The types of psychiatric disorders
seen in the epileptic children and those from the general population
were quite similar.

The Isle of Wight survey suggested that the high rate of psychiatric
disorders in the epileptic children is attributable to the presence of brain
dysfunction rather than simply being the result of a physical handicap
(although this also plays a part). The presence of epilepsy is taken as
evidence of brain dysfunction. Children with other types of brain
dysfunction, including cerebral palsy, low IQ, and reading impairment,
also have higher rates of psychiatric disorders than controls. Most of
the psychiatric disorders seen in the Isle of Wight epileptic children
were similar to the psychiatric disorders seen in the children from the
general population. This study thus suggests a connection between
brain dysfunction of various sorts and psychiatric disorders.

A number of reasons in addition to brain dysfunction have been
advanced to explain the higher incidence of psychiatric problems in the
physically and mentally handicapped (Graham and Rutter, 1968). These
include (1) the reduced ability of mentally handicapped people to
respond to stress, (2) perceptual, speech, and language impairments,
(3) the visible nature of many handicaps, which brings attention to the
handicapped person, (4) the frustration caused by physical restrictions,
and (5) the negative reactions of families to the stresses of having a
handicapped child. These factors, in varying combinations, may result
in behavior or emotional problems.

The high incidence of psychiatric disorders in handicapped
youngsters is an important consideration in their education. Everyone
who provides services to handicapped children and adolescents will
encounter these disorders. The more knowledge the team members

have of psychiatric disorders and of the circumstances that aggravate and relieve these disorders, the more comfortable they will be in working with their clients. If team members can recognize and anticipate the more common behavioral and emotional disorders, these disorders can be treated effectively with the least disruption to the child and to his or her classroom.

Multidisciplinary Care

It is no longer possible for a single person to care for all of the needs of a handicapped child. Rather, a team of specialists from a number of disciplines works together to educate and rehabilitate handicapped children. A child with a single handicap, whether it is blindness, deafness, or paralysis, will have special educational and psychosocial needs at the very least. Other children, depending on their handicaps, will also need occupational, physical, speech, or psychological services. The more handicapped the child, the more likely the need for multiple services. Ancillary services, such as school bus services and home health assistance, may also be required.

The body of knowledge in many of these specialties is so great that one person is usually able to acquire expertise in only one. If personnel are scarce, occasionally a physical therapist can assume the responsibilities of both physical and occupational therapy. Because the tasks of each specialty frequently do not overlap, however, a therapist acting as a double specialist usually is unable to do a thorough job in both areas. Recognizing this, a specialist will perform a dual role only temporarily. Furthermore, as knowledge about and the numbers of handicapped persons have increased, there has been a tendency to further subdivide service areas to improve care delivery. For example, the specialties of child life and therapeutic recreation have developed in hospitals and have expanded the services that previously were performed by nurses, teachers, and occupational and physical therapists. These specialists, trained in child development, supervise leisure activity and help children adjust to hospital and residential life.

Schools, hospitals, and other agencies need the involvement of many specialists in a multidisciplinary team approach. It is important that decisions about diagnoses and treatment of handicapped children be made and discussed in the presence of all personnel involved in the care of these children. If a decision about a child's care must be made before the team meets, that decision and its ramifications should be discussed later by everyone involved.

It is best when all necessary services for a handicapped child can be carried out in a single agency. With such centralized care, treating personnel can communicate frequently with one another in scheduled meetings and in unscheduled informal exchanges. For example, when the physical therapist transfers a patient to the occupational therapist, the two team members can share worthwhile information. PL 94-142 has resulted in comprehensive centralized care for many handicapped children within the school. Many of these children would previously have not received certain services or would have received services at agencies removed from the school premises.

The multidisciplinary team meeting serves as a forum for discussion at which the observations and opinions of team members are shared. The attendance of everyone involved with the child is important because a specialist who is absent has no input and may receive a distorted impression of what occurred at the meeting. In addition, later on he or she may not understand what is happening during a specific treatment. When the treatment of a handicapped child is shared with other agencies, the chances of disagreement or misunderstanding increase. When a form of treatment is not standardized, therapists working in different agencies may duplicate treatments or may make contradictory suggestions. Families become bewildered when therapies are contradictory, disorganized, or inconsistent. Good communication in a well-organized multidisciplinary team situation can, however, lessen or eliminate such problems.

The multidisciplinary team consists of specialists, administrators, and others who are involved in the care of a group of handicapped youngsters. Multidisciplinary teams vary in their membership, stability, size, function, and the extent of involvement with the handicapped child or adolescent. They may serve in hospitals, schools, vocational settings, or other agencies, and they may be involved with diagnosis, treatment, or a combination of diagnosis and treatment. The team's function determines the length of time that it is involved with a child.

Hospital Teams

Team members in a hospital-based child development center may evaluate a handicapped child over a 3- to 5-day period and then meet to formulate a set of recommendations for schools and other agencies. Aside from a few periodic follow-ups, the function of this type of multidisciplinary team does not extend beyond evaluation.

Another type of team is found on a hospital rehabilitation unit. (See Table 1–3 for the specialties that are represented on a hospital rehabilitation unit team.) This team also evaluates a child over a 1-week period and then meets to formulate the treatment plan which they themselves will carry out. Children's initial treatment plans may cover a period ranging from a week to several months. The team meeting to decide on the child's treatment plan is followed by a meeting between team

TABLE 1–3.
Services Represented on a Pediatric Rehabilitation Team

Medical specialties	Psychology
Nursing	Child life/Therapeutic recreation
Nutrition	Social work
Occupational therapy	Special education
Physical therapy	Speech and language
Psychiatry	

members and the parents. At this time the family has the opportunity to discuss the evaluation and the recommendations. Throughout the patient's stay, the multidisciplinary team holds weekly progress meetings and periodic reassessments. At the end of the hospital stay, the team prepares a final assessment and arranges for follow-up visits. If outpatient treatments are necessary, the involved specialist arranges appropriate referrals and confers with outside therapists.

Education Teams

State and local school systems dictate the composition of multidisciplinary teams involved in the evaluation and education of handicapped children. The specialists who evaluate children on their initial referral compose one multidisciplinary team. The specialists who use the evaluations to make appropriate school placements compose another multidisciplinary team, which may also review each child's program yearly. The specialists and administrators in the local school compose the treatment team responsible for carrying out the program constructed by the evaluation and placement teams. The treatment team meets regularly to discuss the student's educational plan, to modify the plan if necessary, and to provide feedback to the review team. When outside agencies are involved with handicapped children and adolescents, it is important that their input be delivered to the school treatment and review teams to best serve the child. The education team and its work is discussed in greater detail in Chapters 6 and 7.

Mental Health Teams

The mental health team may be part of a larger evaluating or treating team within a school or agency, or it may be a separate group located within a hospital or a mental health clinic. Specialists concerned with mental health issues include psychiatrists, psychologists, social workers, mental health professionals, and psychiatric nurses. The size and membership of the mental health team will vary depending on the mental health needs of the facility and whether the team is a separate entity or part of another, larger team. For example, the mental health team in a physical therapy agency may consist of a single social worker who deals with most problems that arise with clients and who makes only an occasional referral to a psychiatrist. By contrast, the mental health team in a school for emotionally disturbed children may include a psychiatrist, a behavioral psychologist, a cognitive psychologist, and several social workers.

Referral and Definition of Problems

Behavioral, emotional, and family problems that impede educational and therapeutic progress are brought to the attention of psychiatrists or psychologists. These problems often are obvious. A team member may notice that a particular child is doing something different or peculiar but cannot identify the behavior as being a psychological impairment. The team member can, however, describe how this particular behavior is preventing educational advancement. When he or she brings the behavior to the attention of the multidisciplinary team, other members may describe similar troublesome behaviors. Together group members discuss and amplify the description of the noted behavior. It is an advantage to have the mental health team member who originally assessed the psychological status of the child involved in this discussion because this person can contribute his or her initial impression as a baseline comparison for the current situation. The mental health specialist can help to define the psychological problems that prevent educational progress.

A psychiatrist or psychologist can also review a treatment course that is proving unsatisfactory and may discover a psychological component that is not apparent without expert scrutiny. For example, an emotional disorder in a parent may impede a child's progress when all other components of the educational plan appear to be working well. Sometimes it may take months or years of interaction with a family before such an emotional problem is identified. The child described in the following case history received several evaluations before the primary role of his mother's mental illness was clarified.

Doug was a 6-year-old kindergarten student evaluated at a child development center for a long history of behavior problems and poor school performance. Sleep and eating patterns had been irregular, and activity level had been high since infancy. Doug showed perseveration on tasks that interested him. Tantrum behavior appeared at age 2 years. He also began to show aggressive behavior to his mother and his 9-year-old sister. The kindergarten school teacher stated that Doug was immature and appeared to be unhappy at times, and school testing revealed normal intelligence but poor performance ability. The parents decided to have Doug repeat kindergarten in another school. At the same time they took him to a mental health clinic for evaluation of hyperactivity and aggressive behavior. Methylphenidate (Ritalin) was prescribed but was discontinued after a week because Doug developed stomachaches and became more talkative. The psychiatrist then prescribed pemoline (Cylert), which made the child more active. He next prescribed imipramine, which decreased the child's activity level but caused fatigue and irritability. The parents discontinued the imipramine.

The developmental evaluation demonstrated above-average intellectual resources without evidence of learning disability. Separation anxiety was evident during evaluations by different team members. Doug habitually bit his fingernails and had a history of lip biting. There was no evidence of the presence of attentional disorder. The psychiatrist noted that the child became sad and anxious when his mother was discussed, and Doug told the examiner that his mother was sad and cried a lot. He said he could sometimes cheer her up by helping her mop. Individual therapy was recommended for both the child and his parents. His father disagreed with the evaluation report in a written letter to the center. Two months after the evaluation, Doug's father phoned the psychiatrist requesting a psychiatric referral for his wife. She had developed agitated behavior and was subsequently arrested for attempting to assault a policeman. She chose to enter a psychiatric hospital, where manic-depressive illness was diagnosed and treated. After her acute hospitalization, the mother attended outpatient therapy, where her therapist focused on parenting skills, including her discipline and her interactions with both of her children. Doug's school performance and home behavior improved during this period.

Discovery of the mother's mental illness as a major reason for her son's emotional disturbance led to a different focus of treatment and subsequent improvement in the child.

Mental Health Team Members

CHILD PSYCHIATRISTS. The child psychiatrist provides leadership for the mental health team. The child psychiatrist is both a medical doctor and a mental health specialist, and as a physician he or she uses a medical approach to evaluation of symptoms and diagnosis of illness. The medical approach consists of a careful history followed by examination of the patient. Child psychiatrists often use tests or special procedures to assist them in reaching the diagnosis, which determines subsequent treatment. Treatments the psychiatrist may employ include drug treatment, psychotherapy, and psychosocial treatments. A more detailed discussion of medical treatment of psychiatric disorders in handicapped children is found in Chapter 4.

Medical diagnosis is more difficult in child psychiatry than in pediatrics because there are fewer visible signs and few laboratory tests that clearly distinguish between one illness and another. For example, the pediatrician can diagnose certain tumors by history, examination, and CT scan. However, the child psychiatrist must rely on verbal reports and subjective observations to reach a diagnosis. The reliability of informants thus becomes an important consideration. The adoption and widespread use by psychiatrists of the American Psychiatric Association's Diagnostic and Statistical Manual, Third Edition (DSM III) (1980), now revised as DSM III-R (1987), is an important step toward increasing diagnostic accuracy by creating standards for diagnosis. When using this manual, a psychiatrist must identify a specific number of criteria to give a patient a certain diagnosis.

As a mental health specialist, the child psychiatrist has had at least 4 years of training beyond medical school in the diagnosis and treatment of patients with mental disorders. He or she is familiar with the main theories of normal and abnormal development and personality and has worked with outpatients and inpatients suffering from a range of illnesses, from minor problems of adjustment to major mental illnesses. The child psychiatrist is also able to contribute to the diagnosis of retardation, language disorders, and brain damage.

In diagnosing a child's disorder, the psychiatrist first obtains a history from the parents and then evaluates the child through observation, conversation, and play. He or she also obtains corroborating material from schools and other involved facilities and input from other team members. The psychiatrist then prepares a written diagnostic evaluation and presents his or her impression and recommendations at the multidisciplinary team's evaluation conference. If the psychiatrist is a consultant, treatment recommendations are implemented by staff mental health workers. If the psychiatrist is a staff member, he or she may become the therapist or participate in the therapy—for example, by prescribing and following medication usage.

Community and child mental health centers may have one or more psychiatrists on their staffs, as may larger agencies and hospital facilities. Child psychiatrists generally serve as consultants to schools or agencies. In some settings psychologists or social workers rather than psychiatrists may be responsible for evaluation and treatment of behavioral and emotional disorders. These mental health personnel have become qualified to use the guidelines of the DSM III-R psychiatric manual when they evaluate their patients. The coding system of this manual is used by government and insurance third-party payers when claims for psychiatric reimbursement are evaluated.

PSYCHOLOGISTS. Clinical psychologists frequently serve on mental health teams. These specialists have completed graduate training in areas of normal and abnormal psychology and have had clinical experience with a range of emotional and behavioral disorders. Clinical psychologists evaluate and treat patients using a variety of treatment methods. One type of clinical psychologist, the behavioral psychologist, analyzes maladaptive behaviors and then constructs treatments based on methods of operant and classical conditioning (see Chapter 5). Cognitive and/or educational psychologists provide a wide variety of testing services, including intelligence and aptitude tests. Tests must be constructed or adapted to serve special populations, such as blind, deaf, and learning disabled children. Results of these tests provide useful information to special educators and psychotherapists.

A neuropsychologist is a person whose services are important in certain cases. This specialist, an expert in evaluation and treatment of patients with brain damage, creates and administers tests that define motor, cognitive, and psychological deficits in terms of specific impairment of brain function. More recently, neuropsychologists have helped to devise programs of cognitive remediation for children and adolescents who have suffered traumatic brain injuries.

SOCIAL WORKERS. The social worker is an indispensable member of the mental health team. The tasks of social workers are multiple and vary according to the needs and philosophy of the facility at which they are employed. Some social workers work to achieve the best possible living, academic, and vocational situations for clients and their families. Some social workers work with families of handicapped children to improve their adjustment with respect to social and economic functioning. Still other social workers are engaged as psychotherapists for the child and/or family members. If the social worker's caseload is small, he or she will be able to direct a great deal of attention to the needs of individual children and their families. Large caseloads, of course, dictate a more limited involvement. Chapter 8, written by a social worker, explores issues of concern to these professionals as they work with the families of handicapped children.

CASE MANAGERS. As the number of services for handicapped children proliferates, the need for coordination of services increases so that they will work well for children and their families. This need for coordination is most apparent when services for a multiply handicapped child are divided among a number of agencies. In these situations a case manager is needed. He or she helps families understand their child's and their own needs, evaluate suggested therapies, plan a schedule for all necessary services, and measure therapeutic progress.

A case manager is a professional who coordinates the child's and family's needs with all of the services being provided. The more services and agencies involved, the more important the role of the case manager. Various specialists may be designated to fill this role. Often the member of the multidisciplinary team who provides a major service to the patient will volunteer to be the case manager. For example, the physical therapist might be the case manager for a child with severe spastic diplegia, or the speech and language pathologist might be the case manager for a dysphasic child. It is assumed that the personnel mentioned are most knowledgeable and therefore most effective in solving problems concerned with the deficits in their particular clients. When the paramount concern is the coordination of services among agencies and the family, the social worker often is a logical choice for the case manager position. He or she is knowledgeable about resources and is skilled in securing and maintaining services for families who need them. Other opinions concerning qualifications for a case manager include the need for an active advocacy component. An important factor to be aware of when choosing a case manager is that it is time consuming, and the manager needs sufficient time to perform the role well.

OTHER MENTAL HEALTH TEAM MEMBERS. Other professionals may participate on the mental health team. These include mental health professionals, psychiatric nurse practitioners, psychiatric nurses, and a variety of specialized counselors. These specialized counselors may staff programs dedicated to alcohol and drug abuse prevention, suicide prevention, or education about sex and pregnancy.

SUMMARY

Since passage in 1975 of PL 94-142 (The Education for All Handicapped Children Act), the public school system has assumed leadership in providing education and rehabilitation services for handicapped children and adolescents. The evaluation and treatment of such youngsters is a multidisciplinary effort, performed by specialists from various disciplines. Because the incidence of psychiatric disorders is very high in handicapped children and adolescents, it is important that all professionals who work with such youngsters be able to recognize potential emotional or behavioral problems. The mental health members of the multidisciplinary team are equipped to discuss in detail the problems presented by other team members and then to offer treatment suggestions. In multidisciplinary team settings, team members discuss the major physical and mental handicaps that impair a child's learning. In addition, the behavioral and emotional problems that children display will significantly influence the team's treatment decisions.

REFERENCES

Abramowicz, H.K., and Richardson, S.A. (1975). Epidemiology of severe mental retardation in children: Community studies. *American Journal of Mental Deficiency, 80,* 18–39.

American Association on Mental Deficiency. (1983). *Classification in mental retardation.* Washington, DC: Author.

American Psychiatric Association. (1980). *Diagnostic and statistical manual* (3rd ed.). Washington, DC: Author.

American Psychiatric Association. (1987). *Diagnostic and statistical manual* (3rd ed.)—revised. Washington, DC: Author.

Brannon, J.B., and Murray, T. (1966). The spoken syntax of normal, hard-of-hearing, and deaf children. *Journal of Speech and Hearing Research, 9,* 604–610.

Breslau, N., Staruch, K.S., and Mortimer, E.A. (1982). Psychological distress in mothers of disabled children. *American Journal of the Diseases of Childhood, 136,* 682–686.

Chess, S., and Hassibi, M. (1970). Behavior deviations in mentally retarded children. *Journal of the American Academy of Child Psychiatry, 9,* 282–297.

Fraiberg, S., and Fraiberg, L. (1979). *Insights from the blind: Comparative studies of blind and sighted infants.* New York: New American Library.

Graham, P., and Rutter, M. (1968). Organic brain dysfunction and child psychiatric disorder. *British Medical Journal, 3,* 695–700.

Gualtieri, C.T., Koriath, U., VanBourgondien, M., and Saleeby, N. (1983). Language disorders in children referred for psychiatric services. *Journal of the American Academy of Child Psychiatry, 22,* 165–171.

Horton, K.B. (1974). Infant intervention and language learning. In R.L. Schiefelbusch and L.L. Lloyd (Eds.), *Language perspectives: Acquisition, retardation, and intervention* (pp. 468–491). Baltimore: University Park Press.

Kakalik, J.S., Brewer, G.D., Dougharty, L.A., Fleischauer, P.D., and Genensky, S.M. (1973). *Services for handicapped youth: A program overview.* Santa Monica, California: Rand Corporation.

Martin, E.W. (1985). Pediatrician's role in the care of disabled children. *Pediatrics in Review, 6,* 275–281.

Matkin, N.D. (1984). Early recognition and referral of hearing-impaired children. *Pediatrics in Review, 6,* 151–156.

Menolascino, F. (1971). Psychiatric aspects of retardation in young children. In R. Koch and J.C. Dobson (Eds.), *The mentally retarded child and his family: A multidisciplinary handbook* (pp. 386–419). New York: Brunner/Mazel.

Nelson, K.B., and Ellenberg, J.H. (1986). Antecedents of cerebral palsy: Multivariate analysis of risk. *New England Journal of Medicine, 315,* 81–86.

Nelson, L.B. (1984). The visually handicapped child. *Pediatrics in Review, 6,* 173–182.

Niederland, W.G. (1980). Narcissistic ego impairment in patients with early physical malformations. In J. Gliedman and W. Roth (Eds.), *The unexpected minority: Handicapped children in America* (pp. 518–534). New York: Harcourt Brace Jovanovich.

Reid, A.H. (1980). Psychiatric disorders in mentally handicapped children: A clinical and follow-up study. *Journal of Mental Deficiency Research, 24,* 287–298.

Resnick, T.J., Allen, D.A., and Rapin, I. (1984). Disorders of language development: Diagnosis and intervention. *Pediatrics in Review, 6,* 85–92.

Simeonsson, R.J., Cooper, D.H., and Scheiner, A.P. (1982). A review and analysis of the effectiveness of early intervention programs. *Pediatrics, 69,* 635–664.

Stanley, F.J. (1982). An epidemiological study of cerebral palsy in Western Australia, 1956–1975: III. Postnatal aetiology. *Developmental Medicine and Child Neurology, 24,* 575–585.

Szymanski, L.S. (1977). Psychiatric diagnostic evaluation of mentally retarded individuals. *Journal of the American Academy of Child Psychiatry, 16,* 67–87.

The Upton School (1984). *Home and Hospital Services: Policies and programs.* Baltimore: The Upton School.

Wright, G.F. (1982). The pediatrician's role in Public Law 94–142. *Pediatrics in Review, 4,* 191–197.

CHAPTER 2

DESCRIBING AND DIAGNOSING PSYCHIATRIC CONDITIONS IN HANDICAPPED CHILDREN

Joan P. Gerring

The term handicap implies that a physical, cognitive, or psychiatric problem has been diagnosed. A child may have one or more diagnoses; that is, a problem may exist by itself, or it may coexist with other problems. This coexistence is sometimes called "dual diagnosis," and it may complicate the diagnostic and therapeutic processes in ways that are discussed in this chapter. This chapter begins with a description of psychiatric classification, and then describes the process of evaluating patients. Finally, psychiatric symptoms and disorders that are commonly found in handicapped youngsters are considered.

THE NEED TO CLASSIFY PSYCHIATRIC CONDITIONS

Children exhibit a wide variety of psychiatric problems. These problems must be defined clearly so that all involved professionals understand them and can converse with each other about them. Clear communication is especially challenging and important when professionals from several specialties are involved in the care of a child, which is usually the situation when handicapped children have psychiatric problems. For example, the special educator and the physical therapist may describe a child's behavior that is interfering with his or her progress, using language that is familiar to them. These two specialists must come to understand each other's perceptions of the child and the problem. The psychiatric system of classification of mental disorders can be of help to them.

When a psychiatrist is consulted on a case, he or she evaluates the child and, using psychiatric terms, defines the child's disorder and presents evidence for it to the referring professionals. These professionals then have the opportunity to present their perceptions of the child's behavior and to support or disagree with the psychiatrist's impression. This discussion facilitates communication and consensus among the psychiatrist and the treating professionals. The psychiatrist then offers treatment recommendations in the interdisciplinary fashion outlined in Chapter 1.

Developing a classification system of mental disorders in psychiatry has been difficult. Many different kinds of professionals are involved with the clinical study and treatment of mental disorders, and each discipline views these disorders in a different way. In fact, even within psychiatry there are differences of opinion about how to define particular disorders. With this in mind, psychiatrists in the United States have paid great attention to the creation of the present diagnostic system, a system that defines over 200 psychiatric disorders.

This classification system, called Diagnostic and Statistical Manual III–Revised (DSM III-R) (American Psychiatric Association, 1987) is an improvement over previous, more general classification systems. DSM III-R was designed to be comparable to the Ninth Revision of the International Classification of Diseases (ICD-9), a World Health Organization classification of disease used throughout the world. DSM III-R names, describes, and defines each of the mental disorders with specific operational criteria. These are the clinical features that must be present if a diagnosis is to be made. DSM III-R does not speculate about the causes of the disorders, nor does it recommend treatment. The DSM III-R system is not considered final; it will be revised as research findings add to what is now known about mental disorders.

Reliability, or diagnostic agreement among clinicians, is a goal of a good classification system. That is, a child should receive the same psychiatric diagnosis from any psychiatrist who evaluates him or her. Validity is another goal. Validity refers to the accuracy of the descriptions of particular disorders. Valid categories of disorders are hard to achieve because in child psychiatry there is not yet a great deal of information about the histories of these disorders and their family patterns (Cantwell, 1980).

THE EVALUATION PROCESS

If the focus of the psychiatric evaluation is placement in special education, the evaluation must demonstrate the presence of a mental disorder that constitutes a handicap to the child's learning. That is, the psychiatrist must demonstrate that the mental disorder is contributing significantly to the child's poor academic performance. Sometimes a mental disorder has little measurable effect on the child's learning.

Because children do not often complain of psychological distress, they are usually referred by parents or other adults for evaluation of home or school problems. Children may not agree that there is a problem, or they may not understand the nature of the problem. They may not cooperate with the evaluation. Moreover, the child's participation in the evaluation may be limited by age or cognitive or language limitations. Even if children are cooperative, they may have trouble describing their emotional states or reactions. Many methods, such as play therapy, drawing, and game playing, have been developed to elicit information about the emotional conflicts and reactions of the nonverbal child. Despite these methods, emotional states and misbehaviors reported by parents or teachers often do not appear during the structured interview with the child.

Because children cannot be relied on to report or demonstrate their psychiatric problems, parent interviews and school reports are necessary parts of the evaluation process. In fact, Graham and Rutter (1970) found the interview with the parents to be the most useful method in detecting psychiatric disorder. If the parents report no evidence of mental disorder in their child, and the school reports no disorder, it is unusual for the psychiatrist to detect disorder in the interview with the child.

Thus, it is important that the child and his or her parent(s) be present and that school information be available at the time of the evaluation. The psychiatrist's impressions, diagnoses, and treatment recommendations will be valuable only if these information sources are complete and accurate.

Psychiatric evaluations most often occur in a single session lasting 1 to 2 hours. Children and their parents may be interviewed separately or together. How the interview is managed varies according to the practice of the psychiatrist and the particularities of the situation. The parent may be asked to give a history of the child's problem and development while the child remains in the waiting room. Then the child is interviewed. A teenager is sometimes interviewed first to help establish a better initial rapport. It is always helpful for the psychiatrist to see the patient and parent together in order to observe the parent-child interaction. In evaluating children with severe limitations, the psychiatrist may interview parents and children together because children with limited intellect or social skills sometimes communicate best when they are with their parents. In addition, the parent can be asked to demonstrate special skills or behaviors that the psychiatrist does not know about or cannot elicit from the child.

Some children cannot be left unattended in the waiting room while the parent is being interviewed because they are too young, too handicapped, or too disruptive. In such cases, if it is possible, more than one family member should attend the interview to provide information and to assist in care of the child. Some evaluation centers provide child life specialists who attend to patients and their siblings in a play room setting while parents are being interviewed. These child life professionals often can provide valuable information to the psychiatrist about how the patient interacts with siblings and others.

The Parent Interview

As already stated, the interview with the parents is the best way to detect psychiatric disorder in the child. Thus, the psychiatrist must know how the parents view the evaluation. Parents may refer the child themselves, or they may agree with the referring professionals that their child has a psychiatric problem. On the other hand, some parents do not agree that there is a problem. To ensure parents' cooperation, it is important to discuss with them the purpose and goals of the evaluation.

The psychiatrist begins the interview by asking the parents to describe the child's problem. They are given time to describe this problem (or lack of problem) in their own words, uninterrupted by questions. The psychiatrist then asks questions about the problem and associated behaviors and emotions needed to make a diagnosis. For example, a child may be referred for stealing school property. In addition to obtaining details of this and any previous thefts, the psychiatrist asks about other examples of misbehavior, such as running away and lying. In this way the psychiatrist investigates the possibility of a diagnosis of conduct disorder.

Whatever the present problem, the psychiatrist inquires about the possibility of other behavioral and emotional disorders. All aspects of their child's mental and physical functioning are discussed with the parents, with special attention being given to the child's assets. The psychiatrist also assesses the emotional, social, and economic functioning of the family. A family psychiatric history is included in the evaluation, because many mental disorders have a hereditary component. If family psychiatric disorder is detected, further assessment will be directed to this area.

The Child Interview

The interview with the child is the central feature of the evaluation and always yields important information. The amount and type of information varies according to the child's ability to communicate and to the kind of psychiatric problem that he or she is presenting. When the child is handicapped, the psychiatrist gets additional information and insight from their meeting. Observation may be all that is possible with some children who have severe intellectual or language impairment or with children who show extreme social aloofness. Others may exhibit behaviors, such as aggression, self-stimulation, or hyperactivity, that prevent meaningful interaction between the patient and the examiner. For example, the initial meeting with 5-year-old Marvin, which follows, illustrates problems that may occur in the evaluation interview.

> Marvin was a 5-year-old boy who lived with his mother, but who visited his father every day. He was referred by his kindergarten teacher for disruptive classroom behavior. The teacher reported that Marvin did not pay attention, was very active, and frequently disrupted the 22-member class. Marvin was also occasionally aggressive toward his peers.
>
> Marvin and his mother entered the psychiatrist's office for the evaluation. Marvin, an attractive, neatly dressed child, immediately moved from one object to the next, touching, pulling, and rearranging. He had no regard for safety. pulling on heavy objects that could fall on him. He opened desk drawers and took out their contents, disregarding his mother, who told him to sit down. When the psychiatrist asked him to stop touching things, he complied for a short time and then resumed his activity.
>
> It was difficult to get information from the mother or to carry on a conversation with Marvin. There was no provision for child care in the clinic, so there was no opportunity to obtain a history from the mother without Marvin being present. The mother was given a school behavior checklist for the teacher to fill out and was asked to return by herself the next week. In her next meeting with the mother, without Marvin present, the psychiatrist was able to obtain an uninterrupted history and also to get from her the school checklist with its important information.

Throughout the evaluation session, the psychiatrist works to form an impression of what is wrong with the child and to develop ideas about treatment. If, for example, a 10-year-old girl who has been referred for starting fights at school tells the psychiatrist that she never starts the fights and is never to blame, the psychiatrist views the child as lacking insight into her own behavior. The psychiatrist then considers treatment methods that do not rely on the child's ability to profit from interpretation of conversation or play. Rather, a behavioral treatment based on rewards for good behavior, combined with parent counseling, might be a better way to work with this child. However, a 10-year-old boy who describes continued sadness and frequent stomachaches a year following the death of his grandfather would be treated quite differently. This child's conversation and emotional responses might lead the psychiatrist to recommend a talk-based therapy that provides support, clarification, and interpretation.

Often there are several treatments that might be chosen for a particular disorder. Because there are few studies that demonstrate conclusively the superiority of one form of treatment over another, psychiatrists consider several factors when they make treatment recommendations. These include the diagnosis, the characteristics of the child and family, the psychiatrist's own clinical experience and orientation, and the family's financial status.

SCHOOL INFORMATION. School information is very important to psychiatrists as they evaluate children. Handicapped children must use all of their resources to function well in school, and school is often stressful to children who are deficient in academic or social skills. During the course of the school year, teachers see children at their best and their worst. Furthermore, they have an objective view of children that parents often lack, and they can compare the academic and social functioning of a particular child with other children they have taught.

Sometimes parents resist obtaining school input for their child's evaluation. They may not want the school to know that their child is receiving counseling, or they may fear a breach of confidentiality. Conflict between the parent and the school about how the child should be managed is of concern to the psychiatrist. This conflict is a problem particularly when the child is aware of it and participates in it. It is, therefore, important that such situations be clarified at the onset of the psychiatric evaluation.

In evaluating a child's school behavior and performance, the psychiatrist often finds behavior rating scales helpful. Teachers observe the child over a period of time and then fill out a scale that comments on the frequency of certain classroom behaviors. Academic performance may also be described. These scales are usually easy to understand and take only a short time to complete. Space is also available for the teacher to make additional comments about the student. The Child Behavior Checklist Teacher's Report Form (Edelbrock and Achenbach, 1984) is an example of a behavior rating scale that is useful in the evaluation process. Other scales are useful in following specific types of treatment. The Teacher Questionnaire (Conners, 1969) is an example of such a scale (see Figure 2–1). The teacher is asked to evaluate 28 behaviors related to high activity level, impulsivity, and inattention. The teacher completes the scale as part of the psychiatric evaluation and then periodically repeats the scale during therapy to assess treatment effects.

LABORATORY TESTS. Currently, there are no laboratory tests to confirm psychiatric diagnoses. Laboratory tests may confirm the

FIGURE 2-1. Teacher Rating Scale

Name of Child _____ Grade _____

Date of Evaluation _____

Please answer all questions. Beside each item, indicate the degree of the problem by a check mark (✔)

	Not at all	Just a little	Pretty much	Very much
1. Restless in the "squirmy" sense.				
2. Makes inappropriate noises when he shouldn't.				
3. Demands must be met immediately.				
4. Acts "smart" (impudent or sassy).				
5. Temper outbursts and unpredictable behavior.				
6. Overly sensitive to criticism.				
7. Distractibility or attention span a problem.				
8. Disturbs other children.				
9. Daydreams.				
10. Pouts and sulks.				
11. Mood changes quickly and drastically.				
12. Quarrelsome.				
13. Submissive attitude toward authority.				
14. Restless, always "up and on the go."				
15. Excitable, impulsive.				
16. Excessive demands for teacher's attention.				
17. Appears to be unaccepted by group.				
18. Appears to be easily led by other children.				
19. No sense of fair play.				
20. Appears to lack leadership.				
21. Fails to finish things that he starts.				
22. Childish and immature.				
23. Denies mistakes or blames others.				
24. Does not get along well with other children.				
25. Uncooperative with classmates.				
26. Easily frustrated in efforts.				
27. Uncooperative with teacher.				
28. Difficulty in learning.				

Reprinted with permission from Conners, C.K.: A teacher rating scale for use in drug studies with children. *American Journal of Psychiatry* 126: 884-888, 1969.

presence of neurological conditions that can help the psychiatrist diagnose and treat associated psychiatric disorders, however. For example, psychiatric problems are common after severe closed head injury. A CT scan taken as part of a psychiatric evaluation may demonstrate a decrease in the amount of brain substance, confirming that a brain abnormality is present. This important neurological information may help the psychiatrist diagnose associated psychiatric disorders such as dementia or organic personality disorder. Other conditions diagnosable by CT scan that have associated psychiatric disorders include central nervous system tumors and hydrocephalus.

Electroencephalograms (EEGs) are useful in the diagnosis and treatment of children with epilepsy. Many children with psychiatric problems, with and without epilepsy, also have EEG abnormalities. For example, one study reported 50 percent of hyperactive children had abnormal EEGs (Millichamp et al., 1968). It was earlier hoped that aggression, temper tantrums, and other misbehaviors, when accompanied by abnormal EEGs, might be responsive to therapy with anticonvulsants. It was thought that these behaviors might be evidence of seizure-like activity occuring in the brain. Treating children with psychiatric problems and EEG abnormalities with the anticonvulsant phenytoin (Dilantin) has not proved effective, however (Looker and Conners, 1970). Other studies have shown beneficial effects with another anticonvulsant, carbamazepine (Tegretol), on mood, irritability, and impulsive violence in children who have abnormal EEGs (O'Donnell, 1985).

Intelligence and aptitude tests are other valuable sources of information for the psychiatrist. These tests provide information about the children's general levels of intelligence and school performance. They also give some idea about the child's level of adaptive functioning. If the school can provide test information from previous years, the effect of the current psychiatric problem on school functioning and IQ level can be assessed. Sometimes information can be obtained that helps to predict the outcome of a particular psychiatric problem. For example, autistic children who have the highest IQs have the best overall outcome.

Projective psychologic tests such as the Draw-A-Person and the Thematic Apperception Test are often used by psychiatrists. Controlled studies have found that these tests are not helpful in the diagnosis of childhood mental disorders, however. Differences in test results have been found between children with behavioral disorders and normal children, but the meaning of these test differences cannot be generalized to different groups. Nevertheless, some clinicians believe that beyond the issue of diagnosis, projective tests help them understand the patient in ways that are useful during treatment (Gittelman, 1980).

FACTORS THAT CONTRIBUTE TO THE APPEARANCE OF PSYCHIATRIC DISORDERS

Stress

All children encounter stressful events, which may include school, moving, illness, parental conflict, separation and divorce, and the death of a significant other. Handicapped children encounter these and additional stresses, such as periods of increased dependency, social ostracism, and physical disfigurement.

Stress appears to contribute to the onset of psychiatric symptoms in many people. In one study, about 60 percent of people with mental disorders had experienced a severe stress in the 2 weeks before the beginning of the disorder, as compared to a 20 percent incidence of severe stress in people who did not have mental disorder (Brown and Harris, 1978). It is known that the greater the number of stresses and the more severe the stress, the greater the likelihood that symptoms will develop.

Development

Children's development is an important consideration for psychiatrists. Development refers to the progression over time of biological, cognitive, social, and psychological functions. Developing functions include bladder and bowel control; capacities to work, play, and form friendships; and responsibility for the management of one's body (Freud, 1972). As different functions may develop somewhat independently of one another, a child may function on a higher level in one area than in another. This situation is commonplace and contributes to the wide range of normal human variation. Sometimes an imbalance in the development of various functions may contribute to the development of emotional or behavioral problems.

Psychiatrists must make judgments as to whether behaviors are within a normal developmental range or whether they are evidence of a developmental lag. Some developmental lags, as well as the absence of positive adaptive behaviors, can be considered evidence of disorder (Achenbach, 1980). In addition, certain behaviors may be normal at one stage of development and maladaptive at another stage. Inattention, impulsivity, and hyperactivity are unremarkable behaviors for a 2-year-old, but for a 9-year-old these behaviors are maladaptive. A 2-year-old may be unable to articulate /p/, /b/, and /t/, but consistent failure of a 3-year-old to articulate these sounds constitutes a developmental articulation disorder.

Another consideration for psychiatrists as they evaluate children is that certain mental disorders may vary in their clinical presentation or in their response to treatment, according to the child's developmental level. For example, manic behavior in children includes temper tantrums, destructiveness, and aggressive outbursts, along with other symptoms that are commonly seen in manic adults (Weinberg and Brumback, 1976). Also, if drug treatment is considered, psychiatrists must take into account the pharmacological differences between children and adults, because the response of a child to a certain drug may be different than the response of an older child or adult.

Children's development is influenced by biological and environmental factors. Beneficial biological factors include normal intelligence, good health, and average physical appearance, whereas low intelligence, poor health, and physical malformation are detrimental to a child's development. Beneficial environmental factors include a stable and nurturing family without much discord, sufficient economic means, and a school that encourages optimal academic development. A discordant family, insufficient income to provide necessities, and a school in which the child's special needs are not met are detrimental to the child's development.

Each developmental stage provides children with a new group of stressful circumstances. For example, entry into first grade is an important developmental landmark that presents children with new stresses. The emphasis in first grade shifts from play to work, and children are asked to give up more pleasurable activities and devote their time to learning. This developmental stage proceeds smoothly when children get satisfaction or gratification from doing school work well. Many hazards exist, however. Children may be anxious because they must leave their parents. They may not be ready to master first grade skills because of slow development, mental retardation, or learning disability. Alternatively, they may be hyperactive or inattentive to a degree that interferes with classroom performance. Developmental difficulties like these may signal or contribute to psychiatric disorder.

Temperament

In addition to stress events and developmental progress, temperament is a factor that is important in psychiatric evaluation. Components of temperament have been extensively studied in many populations of normal and handicapped children. Temperament refers to the child's behavioral style of relating to his or her environment, and it is largely an innate attribute. Chess and her colleagues have divided temperament into nine components: activity level, rhythmicity, approach or withdrawal, adaptability, threshold of responsiveness, intensity of reaction, quality of mood, distractibility and attention span, and persistence (Thomas and Chess, 1984). A child is scored as being high, intermediate, or low in each of these nine categories. Children with certain combinations of temperamental components are at increased risk of developing behavioral problems. For example, children with irregular habits of sleep and feeding (rhythmicity), slow acceptance of new people or routines (adaptability), and frequent periods of loud crying (intensity of reaction) are called difficult children and are vulnerable for the development of behavioral problems.

SYMPTOMS OF MENTAL DISORDER

Symptoms are the complaints of distress or disability that are presented to the psychiatrist by the child or parents. *Signs* of a disorder are observable features seen in a patient, such as a sad expression or a facial tic. The psychiatrist's history and ultimate diagnosis is based on these reported or elicited signs and symptoms. The psychiatrist evaluates each symptom according to its appearance, the length of time it has been present, its characteristics, and its course. The symptom or central problem that brings the child to attention is called the *chief complaint*.

A symptom is further described by its severity, its aggravating factors, and the effects of therapy on it. A symptom may be a temporary impairment that is a response to a stressful situation, or it may be a long-lasting impairment that prevents further psychological development. In some cases, a symptom becomes part of a child's personality and is indistinguishable from a personality trait. Once the patient's symptoms have been described, they can be grouped, and mental disorder(s) can then be diagnosed or ruled out according to diagnostic criteria specified in DSM III-R.

Psychiatric symptoms in children may appear in response to changes in their mental or physical states or in their environment. Such symptoms are seen in all children and might include anxiety or sleep impairment or periods of sadness. However, these symptoms are often temporary; they disappear when circumstances change. A symptom can be as short-lived as 1 hour of anxiety before a piano recital or a night of lost sleep owing to worry about the success of a friend's operation. Symptoms may also last longer and still disappear uneventfully. For example, a child may feel sad for several days after the death of a favorite pet, even showing other symptoms, such as poor appetite and poor concentration.

When children's symptoms last and result in persistent distress or disability, however, they may be brought to the attention of a mental health specialist. The length of time a symptom must last before it is considered pathological has been specified for many disorders in DSM III-R. It must be said, however, that many children have long-lasting psychiatric symptoms that never come to professional attention. These problems are tolerated or are handled in some fashion by families and teachers.

The psychiatric symptoms commonly seen in handicapped children and adolescents and which, in certain groupings, constitute DSM III-R diagnostic criteria for mental disorders will now be discussed. This is followed by a discussion of the mental disorders and their treatments.

PSYCHIATRIC SYMPTOMS

Aggression

When children learn to modify and control their aggression, they can use it to master their environment. This process usually occurs as the young child tries out and masters new activities under the influence of an empathic parent.

Aggression becomes a symptom, however, when it no longer benefits children but rather works to their disadvantage. Aggression may be manifested verbally, as when a child shouts or speaks in a hostile tone. Or it may be physical, as when a child fights or has a temper tantrum or destroys a toy. Aggression may be directed toward the self or toward other people, animals, or objects. It may be described as hostility, rage, cruelty, vandalism, or murder.

A number of factors contribute to the development of aggressive symptoms. These factors may be biological. In one study, neurological impairment and a history of severe head injury distinguished child delinquents who committed murder from child delinquents who did not commit murder. Six of the nine children who had murdered in the study had received head injuries resulting in loss of consciousness (Lewis, 1985). Also, aggressive adolescents have shown abnormalities in neuropsychological functioning (McManus, Alessi, Grapentine, and Brickman, 1984).

Factors contributing to the development of aggressive symptoms may also be social. Loeber and Dishion (1983) concluded that the major factor predicting adolescent aggressive behavior was the parenting style that the young child experienced. An indifferent, rejecting, or negative mother and aggressive methods of punishment are positively correlated with adolescent aggressive behavior. Psychological factors also play a role in the development of aggressive symptoms in children. The quantity and quality of aggression varies widely among individuals and may be a function of temperament, with some children being more irritable, negative, and impulsive than others.

There are two types of self-directed aggressive behavior. The first is suicidal ideation, threats, and attempts. All of the reasons for suicide among nonhandicapped youth also exist for the handicapped. In addition, handicapped youngsters may experience such handicap-related feelings as discouragement about the course of therapy, hopelessness about the future, or decreased self-esteem. (See Chapter 3 for a more detailed discussion of adolescent suicide.)

Self-injurious behavior is the second type of self-directed aggression. This type of behavior, most commonly headbanging, may occur for a time in a minority of seemingly normal infants and toddlers, but it is most commonly seen in the presence of developmental disabilities. Retarded and autistic children may injure themselves in chronic and repetitive ways by behaviors such as biting, pinching, self-striking, repeated vomiting, or eating inedible objects. Medical disorders associated with self-injurious behavior include Lesch-Nyhan syndrome, Cornelia DeLange syndrome, otitis media, and contact dermatitis. Self-injurious behaviors can occasionally result in considerable damage, such as blindness or deafness. Also, when patients are engaged in these behaviors, they are unable to benefit from rehabilitation because the self-injury is often so absorbing and time consuming (Association for Advancement of Behavior Therapy Task Force Report, 1982).

Anxiety

Another feeling which all children experience from time to time is anxiety. From infancy through adolescence, the stresses of emotional and physical changes result in anxiety. These feelings are related to specific phases of development and may even be beneficial as the child works out personal strategies to negotiate each phase. Examples of normal developmental anxieties are the anxiety of the infant about strangers, anxiety connected with performance in primary school, and the anxiety of establishing peer relationships during adolescence.

Anxiety becomes a psychiatric symptom when its presence or its intensity becomes harmful or burdensome to the child. For example, separation anxiety is a type of developmental anxiety experienced by young children as they leave the comfort of home and family. As time goes on, children overcome their distress and derive pleasure from the mastery of being on their own. When separation anxiety intensifies rather than lessens and results in the restriction of a child's activities, a symptom has developed.

The psychiatrist pays attention to both the objective and the subjective components of anxiety in a child. The objective component, what can be observed or measured, includes an appearance of body or facial tension, an increased pulse or blood pressure, and an increased activity level. The subjective component, what patients say they are feeling or what can be inferred about what they are feeling, includes inner tension, apprehension, fearfulness, or dread. Children may describe worry, interrupted sleep, and nightmares. The younger the child or the more cognitively impaired, the more difficult it is to elicit subjective feelings of anxiety. If time is available, children with near normal intelligence can often profit from a general discussion of feeling states before they are questioned about their own feelings. For example, the psychiatrist may describe anxiety to children in terms they can understand and then ask them if they have ever experienced such a feeling.

When anxiety is intense, it is easy to see. When it accompanies other symptoms, such as depression and conduct problems, its presence may not be so apparent. Symptoms of anxiety may also be difficult to distinguish from symptoms of hyperactivity. In such cases, it is necessary to examine the history and other accompanying symptoms to decide which of these two symptoms is present. If tenseness, nail biting, and overeagerness to please accompany the heightened motor activity, the child is likely to have an anxiety disorder. If children are very active for their age and are also inattentive and impulsive but do not show the tenseness or nail biting, they would likely be described as hyperactive. Sometimes anxiety and hyperactivity symptoms coexist, however.

Another way to distinguish between anxiety and hyperactivity is to examine their pattern of occurrence. Anxiety is a symptom that is usually present only in specific situations. Hyperactivity, on the other hand, usually is more pervasive; that is, it occurs in most circumstances. However, this distinction may be difficult to make.

Delusions

Delusions are always a sign of severe disorder, as they indicate a loss of the child's ability to distinguish fantasy from reality. Delusions are false beliefs from which the child or adolescent cannot be swayed. These beliefs or ideas are not shared by members of the child's cultural group. When delusional thinking is suspected, it is important to determine if a close family member is also delusional, for children may develop delusions shared with a delusional parent. Examples of children's delusions are a belief that someone is trying to kill them, a belief that their actions are controlled by an outside force, or the belief that a little man lives inside their stomach and pounds with a hammer to cause pain.

Depression

The feeling of being depressed or unhappy has been experienced by most children and adolescents at one time or another. Depressive mood becomes a psychiatric symptom when it lasts a long time and affects the person in a negative way. Depressive disorders refer to various patterns of depressive symptoms that result in distress and disability. Common characteristics of depressive disorders include sadness, hopelessness, loss of appetite, low self-esteem, irritability, poor concentration, and bodily complaints. Recurrent thoughts of death, suicidal ideas, and suicidal attempts also commonly characterize the thinking of depressed children and adolescents (Pfeffer, Zuckerman, Plutchik, and Mizrucki, 1984).

An earlier view of childhood depression included behaviors that were considered to *mask* underlying depressive feelings. These "depressive equivalents" included hyperactivity, aggressive behavior, bed-wetting, refusal to attend school, and poor school performance. With this older, broader view of depressive symptoms, many children with conduct disorders were viewed as having a "masked depression." The concept of depressive equivalents has been rejected because there was no reliable way to differentiate between children who are, for example, aggressive as a symptom of depression and children who are aggressive as a symptom of a conduct disorder. Moreover, research studies have shown no evidence of an association between depressive mood and symptoms termed "depressive equivalents" (Puig-Antich, 1982b). Rather, a depressive disorder and a conduct disorder may coexist, with conduct disorder symptoms often resolving with antidepressant therapy (Puig-Antich, 1982a).

Symptoms of depression, like those of anxiety, are commonly seen in handicapped children and adolescents as a response to their illnesses and deficits. At each new stage of their development, handicapped children face stressful situations that tax their resources and remind them that they are different. Some of these children react by becoming depressed, developing such symptoms as sadness, decreased concentration, and loss of appetite. For example, symptoms of depression are seen in children following severe traumatic brain injury. These symptoms do not appear until the children have made enough intellectual recovery to be aware of their circumstances. They then become depressed as they become aware of their physical and cognitive handicaps and the social isolation that frequently results from such deficits.

Hallucinations

Hallucinations are perceptions for which there are no identifiable external stimuli. Children may describe hallucinations spontaneously, but more often they have to be asked about them. Most children of normal or low-normal intelligence can distinguish between fantasy and reality. It is sometimes difficult, however, to determine if very young children or retarded children are hallucinating because of their cognitive limitations. Children may at times describe illusions which are misperceptions of real things. For example, they misinterpret the screech of a car as a scream. Careful questioning enables the psychiatrist to distinguish between hallucinations and illusions.

The significance of a hallucination is determined by its characteristics as well as by the symptoms and the situation that accompany it. Voices and visions constitute the majority of hallucinations, although other types, such as taste or smell hallucinations, occasionally occur. Hallucinations may be seen in conditions of deprivation, great anxiety, bereavement, drug ingestion, or brain disorder. A common, often innocent hallucination is the child hearing his or her name called aloud, usually by the parent. Hallucinations may consist of a moral voice, the reassuring voice of an absent parent, or the abusive words of a stern father. A child who is grieving the loss of a loved one may hallucinate the voice or image of that person. At times hallucinations appear to be encouraged by parents because of their own preoccupation with religious experiences or because the child's vision may be beneficial to them. For example, a child's vision of a deceased loved one may help the parents deal with the loss.

Most hallucinations in children are benign or innocent and do not signify serious psychiatric disorder. There is some evidence, however, that children who report benign hallucinations have significantly more relatives with a history of psychotic disorders (Burke, Del Beccaro, McCauley, and Clark, 1985). Sometimes hallucinations are accompanied by other symptoms, such as social isolation, strange beliefs, unusual feelings, or disorganized behavior. The child, at these times, may no longer be able to distinguish between fantasy and reality. These accompanying symptoms lead the psychiatrist to view these hallucinations as symptomatic of a more serious process.

Hyperactivity

Hyperactivity is a common complaint in child psychiatry clinics. This symptom causes disruption in home and school and brings negative attention to the child. A classroom of 25 children can become disorganized with the introduction of a single hyperactive youngster. Such children cannot sit still during a lesson. They fidget in their seats or get up to get something or talk to someone. In this way, other classmates get involved. At home, the parents complain that the child cannot sit still for homework or even for a meal. Hyperactive children disturb their brothers and sisters when they are doing their homework or chores, and at night they sleep restlessly and throw the covers onto the floor.

Most people agree when a child has severe hyperactivity. When the symptoms are less severe, however, differences of opinion occur.

Hyperactivity is a subjective measure. To evaluate this symptom, the psychiatrist relies on information from the parents and the teachers. More objective means of measuring hyperactivity that use a variety of mechanical devices do not have wide clinical usage (Gardner, 1979). Some parents may tolerate and even encourage a high activity level in their child. They may find their very active child less active than an older sibling. Conversely, a parent may label a child with a normal activity level hyperactive. This parent may be unfamiliar with the activity level of children or may not be able to tolerate the activity of a child in the normal range.

Children may be hyperactive all the time, day and night, or they may be hyperactive only in certain situations. Hyperactivity may be more apparent in a structured classroom setting than during a situation of free play, and it may not appear when a child is receiving one-on-one attention.

As with parents, some teachers accept high activity in a child and regard it as a challenge to effectively control the child's behavior. These teachers often regard outside therapeutic intervention as an insult. Yet other teachers seek assistance in managing students who are overly active. They may feel that the extra time needed to manage an overly active child wastes the time of the other students.

Activity level can be a component of temperament. High, intermediate, and low activity levels constitute a range of normal. Again, there is no difficulty in calling severe hyperactivity a psychiatric symptom. Lesser degrees of high activity may be called a feature of temperament, with a different set of treatment suggestions, however. When a child shows high activity, accompanying behaviors help to determine if psychiatric disorder is present.

There is a prominent developmental component to activity level. Young children until age 4 or 5 years may have a high activity level that lessens as they grow. High activity levels become a cause for concern if they persist into grade school. Retarded children may be hyperactive for longer periods, even taking into account their mental age.

Impulsivity

Impulsive children act before they think, and they encounter both school and social problems. These children write or shout out the first answer that comes to mind. They do not think through and organize their school work, and thus close supervision is necessary to ensure that they complete their assignments. When impulsive children play, they cannot wait their turn, and they often interrupt when they are talking with others. Of great concern is the impulsive child's propensity to dart out into the street or to jump out of a window.

Inattention, Distractibility, and Persistence

Inattention and distractibility are psychiatric symptoms that are much alike. Inattention means that the child is unable to remain involved with a task. Distractibility means that various stimuli can easily divert the child's attention from what he or she is doing (Gardner, 1979). These symptoms are similar in that both prevent effective learning and social interaction. Children who cannot keep their minds on their reading assignments are probably not learning the required material. If they are continually distracted by occurrences in the home and classroom, they may not be able to complete their assignments without a lot of supervision. Distracted or inattentive students may also disrupt the work of nearby classmates, and they may not be able to stick to a play activity as well as other children.

Children's attention spans and their degree of distractibility may also be components of their temperaments. Mild, moderate, and high degrees of attention and distractibility can exist within the normal range. Persistence is another feature of temperament that is linked with attention span. Thomas and Chess (1984) describe persistence as the amount of attention adequate to complete a task. It can also be excessive. Great persistence, termed perseveration, is sometimes present in brain injured or mentally retarded children. Perseverative children may be unable to stop an activity when they should. On the other hand, a degree of persistence may be beneficial to handicapped children, enabling them to remain at difficult tasks until they are mastered. It is often difficult for parents to adjust to a very persistent or perseverative child. When the child's persistence is not beneficial, or when accompanying symptoms suggest that a mental disorder is present, the persistence must be investigated further.

Misbehaviors and Conduct Problems

All children misbehave. Handicapped children remain longer in intense dependent relationships with their parents, and they often express their frustrations by misbehaving. Most misbehavior is minor and consists of noncompliance with parents' or teachers' requests. Other misbehaviors include lying, teasing, and provocative and disruptive behaviors. Whining, temper tantrums, and attention-seeking are other misbehaviors that handicapped children may display. These misbehaviors rarely come to professional attention because most of them are minor and short-lived. However, any misbehavior can become a symptom when it becomes too frequent or too intense. An occasional temper tantrum is unremarkable; daily temper tantrums are noteworthy and bear investigation.

Severe misbehaviors usually come to the attention of medical, school, or legal officials. These symptoms may be nonaggressive or aggressive in nature. Nonaggressive conduct problems include truancy, running away, and persistent lying. Any chronic violation of important home, school, or neighborhood rules can constitute a conduct problem if it lasts long enough or is severe enough. Aggressive conduct problems include theft, fire-setting, cruelty to animals, and vandalism. Conduct problems are a handicap to school performance because they are disruptive to the child and his or her classmates, and they take time away from learning. Truancy is an example of a conduct that may lead to great gaps in the child's knowledge. Children with conduct problems may also come to the attention of juvenile authorities, and, in these instances, decisions about education and treatment often become a collaborative effort between the school and the legal system.

Sleep Disturbances

Sleep disturbances are probably universal in childhood. Most disturbances are brief and are related to events or physical states of the previous day. A young child may have a nightmare after a frightening experience or may have restless, interrupted sleep during fever. Another child may be unable to fall asleep after a stimulating birthday party and lots of cola. These disturbances are time-limited and pose little concern.

Other children, however, will have continuing sleep disturbances. The impaired sleep may have a variety of causes, from anxiety to overstimulation to a disorder of the sleep cycle. Parental anxiety often contributes significantly to the clinical picture. The types and frequency of the disturbances vary with the child's stage of cognitive and social development. For example, night waking and reluctance to go to sleep are seen so commonly in 15- to 30-month-old children that they have been regarded as a developmental feature of the age group (Fraiberg, 1950).

Psychiatric sleep symptoms may stem from emotional and physical factors that disturb or disrupt sleep. Emotional aspects include concerns about being alone, fear of the dark, and fear of monsters. Physical aspects include conditions that may disturb sleep; for example, colic, middle ear disease, and certain types of medication (Ferber, 1985). When these emotional and physical factors result in psychological distress or disability, they become symptoms.

In most instances, children's specific sleep impairments can be defined by careful history taking, perhaps including a diary of bedtime events. Sometimes, however, referral of a child to a sleep laboratory is helpful in circumstances under which a serious and remediable disorder of the sleep cycle is suspected. For example, sleep apnea, a condition in which breathing stops for brief periods during the night, can be detected by recording sleep cycles. Narcolepsy, a disorder characterized by frequent episodes of falling asleep during the day, is another condition that can be diagnosed by sleep studies. The affected children spend a night with their sleep waves monitored by EEG wires attached to the scalp. Careful study of the children's sleep behaviors and the EEG record often lead to a diagnosis of the sleep disorder.

MENTAL DISORDERS

Mental disorder is defined as a behavioral or psychological pattern of symptoms that is associated with distress or disability. The disorder can be behavioral, psychological, or biological, but it is not simply a disturbance in social relationships (Spitzer and Cantwell, 1980). The DSM III-R lists some 46 mental disorders or diagnoses that arise or become evident in infancy, childhood, or adolescence. Children or adolescents may also receive diagnoses that are listed in other, adult, sections of the manual. As noted earlier, the clinical features or symptoms are listed for each mental disorder in DSM III-R. The child or adolescent must show a certain number of these features, the diagnostic criteria, before the psychiatrist can make the diagnosis. If information is lacking to reach a definite conclusion, a diagnosis can be deferred until more information becomes available. All possible disorders should be considered, and more than one disorder may be diagnosed in a patient.

There are good reasons to divide mental disorders into two types: behavioral and emotional. Behavioral disorders are observable disturbances of conduct, attention, and activity level. They occur predominantly in males. The families of children with behavioral disorders often show marked discord and may display delinquency, antisocial personality, or drug and alcohol abuse. If a child with behavioral disorder develops a mental disorder in adult life, the disorder is also likely to have antisocial characteristics. In contrast to behavioral disorders, emotional disorders are characterized by internal distress. Emotional disorders are manifested by symptoms such as anxiety, fear, and depression, and boys and girls are affected about equally. Emotional disorders have a better outcome in adolescence and adult life than behavioral disorders. If a child with emotional disorder develops a mental disorder in adult life, the disorder is usually also an emotional disorder (Cantwell, 1980).

To this point symptoms that tend to cluster together have been termed *mental disorders*. However, the term *syndrome* is also frequently used to refer to a group of symptoms. *Disease* is a similar term, used most frequently when referring to physical conditions for which specific biological causes and processes can be identified. When psychiatrists complete their evaluations, they arrive at a diagnosis by matching the child's symptoms to the DSM III-R diagnostic criteria for the most likely disorders.

Two or more disorders often coexist in children. In one survey of 11-year-old children from the general population, the prevalence of mental disorder was 17.6 percent. Fifty-five percent of these disorders occurred in combination with one or more other disorders, and 45 percent occurred as a single disorder (Anderson, Williams, McGee, and Silva, 1987).

Sometimes a mental disorder exists, but the child or adolescent does not fit DSM III-R diagnostic criteria for any disorder, even after extensive information is assessed. For example, disorders of aggressive behavior or disorders of early sexual activity are not yet well described by the current classification system. Certain behavioral disorders of the mentally handicapped, such as extreme self-injury, also need further descriptive work.

Diagnostic uncertainty may be indicated in the following ways. If enough information is present to indicate the class of psychiatric disorder—for example, anxiety—but criteria for a specific anxiety disorder (e.g., generalized anxiety disorder or simple phobia) are not present, the designation of "anxiety disorder, not otherwise specified" (NOS) is given. Also, the designation "(provisional)" may be placed after a specific disorder as an indication of significant diagnostic uncertainty—for example, "generalized anxiety disorder (provisional)."

Sometimes assessment reveals absence of disorder in the child, but there may be family or social conditions that need attention or treatment. Such situations are common and include disturbed relationships between children and parents, isolated antisocial acts, or normal grief reactions. Even when a mental disorder is present, these conditions may be the main focus of treatment. For example, a child with attention-deficit hyperactivity disorder may come for treatment for his or her normal grief reaction following the death of a parent. Alternatively, the treatment may focus on family adjustment to the handicap of a child—for example, adjustment to physical deterioration in an adolescent with muscular dystrophy. The need for classification of family disorders is well recognized, but a reliable system has not yet been developed.

In addition to the diagnosis of mental disorder, the psychiatrist makes qualifying statements in the evaluation that further describe the clinical situation. These statements are in the form of "axes" and are designated by Roman numerals I through V. Each "axis" refers to a different kind of information about the patient and his or her disorder. Axis I is the diagnosis of mental disorders and/or V (vee) codes, conditions other than mental disorders receiving attention. Axis II describes disorders of development or personality; Axis III describes medical conditions the patient may have. Axis IV rates the severity of psychosocial stressors that have contributed to the development, recurrence, or worsening of the patient's mental disorder. Axis V is the psychiatrist's clinical judgment of the patient's current level of academic and social functioning, as well as his or her highest level during the past year. This multiaxial system helps provide a complete medical and psychosocial evaluation of the patient, a clinical picture on which to base treatment planning.

In the following section are discussed several major psychiatric disorders of children and adolescents that are commonly seen in handicapped persons. In the clinical descriptions the aspects of these disorders that are of special importance in handicapped youngsters are emphasized, and current treatment alternatives are discussed. Many of these disorders are considered in further detail in later chapters of this book.

Adjustment Disorder

Adjustment disorder is a common disorder in children and adolescents. The disorder describes a maladaptive reaction to stress that results in impaired social or academic functioning. The disorder must occur within 3 months of the onset of the stress. The diagnosis is not given if the child fulfills criteria for another disorder, such as anxiety or schizophrenia. Adjustment disorder may be manifested by a conduct problem, an emotional disturbance, physical complaints, or a combination of these reactions to stress. For example, a hearing impaired boy may develop provocative behavior and temper tantrums soon after a separation of his parents. Or, an adolescent boy with cerebral palsy may show depression and aggressive behavior after an orthopedic procedure that did not restore his ability to walk. Adjustment disorder should not be viewed as minor because suicidal ideation may be present, and the level of impairment may be high. Adjustment disorder usually abates when the stressful situation stops, and the outlook for full recovery is very good.

Post-traumatic Stress Disorder and Brief Reactive Psychosis

Two other disorders describe children with maladaptive, intense reactions to stressful situations. *Post-traumatic stress disorder* is a response to an extreme stress that is outside the range of usual experience and that would cause symptoms in most people—for example, a kidnapping, an earthquake, or a plane crash. Symptoms include reexperiencing the stress through memories or dreams or repetitive play, avoidance of situations associated with the stress, and development of a pessimistic view about the future. Children may develop symptoms immediately after the stress or after some time has elapsed.

The third disorder that describes reaction to stress is *brief reactive psychosis*. This disorder immediately follows a severe stress and consists of a prominent emotional response accompanied by evidence of psychosis, such as incoherence, hallucinations, and grossly disorganized behavior. The duration of brief reactive psychosis is limited to 1 month.

Brief psychotherapy and pharmacotherapy are used to manage these three stress reactions. Brief psychotherapy should be instituted soon after the appearance of symptoms to provide support for emotional needs and to prevent the development of long-lasting symptoms. The psychiatrist will evaluate intrusive symptoms, such as hallucinations and repeated memories of the stressful event, as well as denial symptoms, such as daydreaming and inattention. The psychiatrist alternately supports and confronts these symptoms to help the child tolerate and better understand the thoughts and emotions connected with the stressful event. The goal is to help the child develop adaptive ways of responding to these thoughts and emotions (Horowitz, 1976). The choice of drug treatment is dictated by the predominant symptoms and the intensity of the reaction.

Anxiety Disorders

Three anxiety disorders in DSM III-R have their onset in childhood or adolescence. Each of these disorders has adult counterparts appearing first after the age of 18 years. One of these, *overanxious disorder*, is a disorder of generalized anxiety. The child worries about many things, is overly concerned about doing well, and is easily embarrassed or humiliated. It is difficult for him or her to relax. Anxiety in the other two disorders occurs only in specific situations. In *avoidant disorder*, the child is anxious in the presence of strangers, and this anxiety restricts the development of peer relationships. The child is not anxious in the presence of familiar people and wants to be socially involved with them.

The anxiety of the third disorder, *separation anxiety disorder*, also focuses on the specific situation of being apart from parents and other significant caregivers. This disorder may take many forms, including school refusal, worry about the well-being of parents, excessive emotional discomfort when leaving parents, and inability to concentrate and perform when parents are away. At times, separation anxiety may be a symptom of childhood depression. The following case history illustrates the clinical picture of a handicapped child who developed a separation anxiety disorder.

Jimmy was the last of five children born into a middle class family. The diagnosis of mild spastic cerebral palsy with speech impairment was made when he was 3 years old. Jimmy entered nursery school at age 3 years and received physical therapy and speech therapy services at school. His adjustment was good, and he entered a regular first grade but continued to receive the special services. During second grade, Jimmy was hospitalized for 1 week for an orthopedic surgical procedure. This was his first period of time away from home. After leaving the hospital, he began to have nightmares and refused to go to sleep without his mother sitting in the room. He resisted the return to school, complaining each morning of a stomachache. After 3 weeks of worsening disturbance, Jimmy's concerned mother brought him for evaluation to the developmental center where he was a patient. The psychiatric consultant diagnosed separation anxiety disorder. Several sessions of play therapy, along with parental counseling, resulted in the disappearance of this acute disorder. Medication can also be effective in the treatment of this disorder.

Panic Disorder, Simple Phobia, and Obsessive Compulsive Disorder

Anxiety is also an important component of three other childhood and adolescent disorders. *Panic disorder* may occur in adolescents. This form of anxiety is composed of discrete attacks of apprehension or fear accompanied by prominent symptoms that include shaking, sweating, chest pain, and difficulty breathing. Some adolescents who develop panic disorder have a history of separation anxiety in childhood.

Anxiety in *simple phobia* is seen as a response to a feared object or situation. Simple phobia consists of an irrational fear, along with a powerful desire to avoid the feared object or situation. The most common childhood phobias are animal phobias.

Obsessive compulsive disorder is another type of anxiety disorder, although it is rare in children. In normal children recurring obsessive thoughts that cannot be put out of mind and compulsive behaviors that children feel they must perform are occasionally seen. Obsessions and compulsions become psychiatric symptoms when children experience them as intrusive and unwanted. They experience anxiety when they attempt to resist the unwanted thoughts and actions. A common adolescent obsession is with recurrent sexual thoughts that are regarded as wrong or sinful. A child is compulsive when, for example, he or she must repeatedly check the position of the slippers under the bed in order to ensure that he or she will be safe during the night.

Psychotherapy has been beneficial in the treatment of anxiety disorders. Psychotherapy is an interaction between therapist and patient that focuses on emotional or behavioral problems and presents alternatives for adaptive change. Behavioral therapy, using techniques of relaxation and desensitization, has resulted in improvement of childhood phobias. Behavioral therapy is a therapeutic interaction that focuses on modification of maladaptive behavior and presents specific prescriptions for change. Antihistamines such as diphenhydramine (Benadryl) and hydroxyzine (Vistaril) and benzodiazepines such as diazepam (Valium) are frequently used for the treatment of childhood anxiety. Controlled studies of treatment results are limited, however. One study has demonstrated the effectiveness of imipramine (Tofranil) in helping children with separation anxiety disorder return to school (Gittelman-Klein and Klein, 1971). Another study has demonstrated the effectiveness of clomipramine, an antidepressant, in the treatment of children with obsessive compulsive disorder (Flament et al., 1985).

Attention-deficit Hyperactivity Disorder

Attention-deficit hyperactivity disorder (ADHD) is a common behavioral disorder with a prevalence of 5 to 10 percent in children and adolescents. The introduction in 1980 in DSM III (American Psychiatric Association, 1980) of the term *attention deficit disorder* (ADD) replaced a number of less precise terms that had previously been used to describe a similar set of behaviors. Persons who have worked many years in the education and treatment of children will recall these commonly used terms (see Table 2–1.) The term *hyperactive reaction of childhood* was the designation used in the 1968 DSM II. Another commonly used term was *minimal brain dysfunction* (MBD). This term implied neurological dysfunction, but it was never strictly defined and was not helpful in making treatment decisions. The indiscriminate use of these different terms in the 1950s and 1960s made clinical studies of attentional problems difficult to interpret.

TABLE 2–1.
Diagnostic Terms That Have Been Replaced by *Attention-Deficit Hyperactivity Disorder*

Hyperactive child syndrome	Minimal brain dysfunction
Hyperkinetic child syndrome	Minimal cerebral dysfunction
Hyperkinetic reaction of childhood	Minor cerebral dysfunction
Minimal brain damage	

The 1980 DSM III definition of attention deficit disorder has undergone further refinement, and in the 1987 DSM III-R the term attention-deficit hyperactivity disorder (ADHD) was introduced. ADHD is defined by criteria of hyperactivity, impulsivity, and inattention. A second disorder, *undifferentiated attention-deficit disorder*, describes individuals with persistent inattention who do not fit into other diagnostic categories. The DSM III-R description of attention-deficit hyperactivity disorder is reproduced here.

Diagnostic Criteria for 314.01 Attention-deficit Hyperactivity Disorder*

Note: Consider a criterion met only if the behavior is considerably more frequent than that of most people of the same mental age.

A. A disturbance of at least 6 months during which at least eight of the following are present:

(1) often fidgets with hands or feet or squirms in seat (in adolescents, may be limited to subjective feelings of restlessness)

(2) has difficulty remaining seated when required to do so

(3) is easily distracted by extraneous stimuli

(4) has difficulty awaiting turn in games or group situations

(5) often blurts out answers to questions before they have been completed

(6) has difficulty following through on instructions from others (not due to oppositional behavior or failure of comprehension), e.g., fails to finish chores

(7) has difficulty sustaining attention in tasks or play activities

(8) often shifts from one uncompleted activity to another

(9) has difficulty playing quietly

(10) often talks excessively

(11) often interrupts or intrudes on others, e.g., butts into other children's games

(12) often does not seem to listen to what is being said to him or her

(13) often loses things necessary for tasks or activities at school or at home (e.g., toys, pencils, books, assignments)

(14) often engages in physically dangerous activities without considering possible consequences (not for the purpose of thrill-seeking), e.g., runs into street without looking

---

*Reprinted with permission from the *Diagnostic and Statistical Manual of Mental Disorders,* 3rd Ed.—revised. Copyright 1987 American Psychiatric Association.

Note: The foregoing items are listed in descending order of discriminating power based on data from a national field trial of the DSM III-R criteria for disruptive behavior disorders.

B. Onset before the age of 7 years.

C. Does not meet the criteria for a pervasive developmental disorder.

Criteria for Severity of Attention-deficit Hyperactivity Disorder

Mild: Few, if any, symptoms in excess of those required to make the diagnosis *and* only minimal or no impairment in school and social functioning.
Moderate: Symptoms or functional impairment intermediate between "mild" and "severe."
Severe: Many symptoms in excess of those required to make the diagnosis *and* significant and pervasive impairment in functioning at home and school and with peers.

ADHD is much more common in boys than in girls and is usually evident by the age of 3 years. A child's heredity plays an important role in the causation of this disorder, although other factors, such as brain injury and seizure disorders, may also play important roles. ADHD is commonly seen in children with mild and moderate mental retardation and learning disabilities. A child living in a disorganized environment may have symptoms of hyperactivity, impulsivity, and inattention indistinguishable from ADHD. In this situation, a detailed psychosocial assessment may sometimes be helpful in making the distinction between the mental disorder of ADHD and a family condition.

The child with ADHD is usually referred to the psychiatrist for evaluation by the parents or the school. The more pronounced the disorder, the earlier the child will be brought to medical attention. Most often the disorder becomes maladaptive upon entry into primary school, where children must be attentive and quiet in order to learn reading and mathematics. The psychiatric evaluation of a child with suspected ADHD begins with a history from the parents and is followed by an interview with the child, in which the psychiatrist may not actually see the symptoms of hyperactivity, inattention, and impulsivity. When the child's examination does not yield useful information, the parents' and the teachers' reports about the child's behavior contribute significantly to the diagnosis. Behavior checklists, such as those described earlier in this chapter, are helpful in obtaining information about a wide range of behaviors.

Although the diagnosis of ADHD comes from the clinical evaluation alone, other examinations and procedures are helpful for comprehensive treatment planning. A complete pediatric evaluation should be performed to rule out remediable causes of impaired attention, such as poor hearing, poor vision, or chronic health problems. Psychometric tests, including intelligence and aptitude tests, provide valuable information about the possible presence of retardation or learning disabilities. A neurological examination may be helpful if a neurological condition such as epilepsy or cerebral palsy is present or suspected. These examinations often demonstrate the presence of motor incoordination and minor neurological abnormalities or immaturities. EEGs, CT scans, and other laboratory procedures, however, have limited usefulness in the diagnosis and treatment of attention-deficit hyperactivity disorder.

Other behavioral and emotional problems frequently occur in children with ADHD. These problems may come directly from the child's symptoms. For example, ADHD children may relate poorly to classmates because they are impulsive and shout out answers or are unable to wait their turn at a game. Or ADHD children may have aggressive outbursts as an impulsive reaction to something that upsets them. As these children grow older, they may develop academic problems after several years of classroom hyperactivity and inattention. The negative responses of others to these children and their poor academic performance are two factors that may lead to decreased self-esteem and depression.

The treatment of ADHD may be pharmacological, behavioral, educational, or a combination of these methods. Psychostimulants, such as methylphenidate (Ritalin), dextroamphetamine (Dexedrine), and pemoline (Cylert), result in significant improvement in 70 to 80 percent of affected children. Ritalin is the most common treatment for ADHD, being widely prescribed by psychiatrists, pediatricians, and general medical practitioners. The optimal dosage schedule for a child is reached by monitoring the drug's effects with the help of the parents and classroom teacher. These drugs result in improved attention, decreased impulsivity, and decreased activity level. It is unknown whether they result in a sustained improvement in learning. When psychostimulants are ineffective, other medications such as antidepressants may be beneficial in the treatment of ADHD.

A comprehensive treatment approach is needed to address the emotional and educational problems that frequently accompany ADHD. The multidisciplinary team often combines medication with educational and behavioral strategies. These strategies may include minimizing distractions, minimizing the impact of attentional deficits, and teaching students how to organize work, material, and time (Shaywitz and

Shaywitz, 1984). Psychotherapy and parent counseling are also useful when the child develops a maladaptive reaction or when the family needs assistance in managing their child. The treatment of attention-deficit hyperactivity disorder is discussed in further detail in Chapters 3, 4, and 6.

Conduct Disorder and Oppositional Defiant Disorder

Conduct disorder is the most common reason for which children and adolescents are referred to psychiatrists. This disorder is defined as the persistent violation of societal rules and the rights of others by young-sters under 18 years of age. Conduct disorder is a psychiatric diagnosis, whereas juvenile delinquency is a legal term. A juvenile delinquent is a child or adolescent under 18 years of age who has committed a crime that would be considered an adult criminal offense, e.g., armed robbery. Some symptoms of conduct disorder constitute such criminal offenses in the legal system, and therefore youngsters who have committed armed robbery or rape, for example, are labeled juvenile delinquent as well as being diagnosed as having conduct disorder. Because the mental health, juvenile justice, and school systems all share an interest in these youngsters, there is need for common understanding and cooperation in managing them.

Aggressive behavior is the most common complaint about children who are being evaluated for conduct disorders. Nine of the 13 DSM III-R diagnostic criteria for conduct disorder are aggressive behaviors. For example, one criterion is that the child often initiates physical fights. Conduct disorder is subdivided into three types. The essential feature of solitary aggressive type, the first type, is aggressive physical behavior. Group type, the second type of conduct disorder, describes conduct problems occurring as a group activity. Undifferentiated type, the third type, includes problems that fulfill criteria for conduct disorder but which do not fit into the other two types. Severity of the disorder is determined by the number of conduct problems and the degree of harm the child inflicts on others.

Other diagnoses frequently accompany conduct disorders. The presence of a second disorder influences the clinical picture and figures prominently in treatment decisions. Attention-deficit hyperactivity disorder is frequently seen in youngsters with conduct disorder, as are depressive disorders. A schizophrenic adolescent may have shown evidence of conduct disorder prior to the onset of a thought disorder, and substance abuse may occur with conduct disorder.

Oppositional defiant disorder describes behavioral symptoms that are less severe than those of conduct disorder. In this disorder, children are defiant and provocative toward authority figures, and they misbehave in this way considerably more frequently than most youngsters of the same mental age. Their symptoms include blaming others, frequently losing their temper, being easily annoyed by others, and refusing to comply with parental requests. If oppositional defiant behavior is seen as part of a psychotic or a depressive disorder, the diagnosis of oppositional defiant disorder is not given.

There are children with behavioral symptoms who do not fit into diagnoses such as attention-deficit hyperactivity disorder, conduct disorder, or oppositional defiant disorder. This is a common problem with the present classification system. For example, retarded children frequently have periods of maladaptive behavior that do not fit the criteria for currently defined disorders. Such instances of behavior may be placed in a nonspecific diagnostic category, e.g., depressive disorder not otherwise specified, or may be called unspecified mental disorder (nonpsychotic), but they should be described carefully by the psychiatrist. Some retarded children with a specific pattern of severe behavioral and/or emotional disturbances are given the diagnosis of pervasive developmental disorder, not otherwise specified.

Conduct disorder is a complicated and poorly understood condition. Treatments using psychological, social, behavioral, and medical methods have had limited success. These treatment methods, used alone or in combination, include individual or group therapy (or both), behavior therapy, parenting skills training, and inpatient milieu therapy. Children with more severe conduct disorders are often sent to residential treatment centers and juvenile detention centers.

Because of the difficulty of treating conduct symptoms successfully, the evaluating psychiatrist must search for the presence of accompanying disorders that may be more amenable to treatment. For example, if a child has attention-deficit hyperactivity disorder or is depressed, the treatment of these disorders may lead to a lessening of the conduct problems that brought the child to the psychiatrist's attention in the first place. When evaluating children with flagrant conduct symptoms, psychiatrists may feel pressured by other professionals to label these children speedily as conduct disordered and move them to another situation. They must resist this pressure, however, and thoroughly search for remediable symptoms, reviewing the child's past history and old records and interviewing people as they seek to shed new light on the case.

Major Depressive Episode, Bipolar Disorder, and Dysthymia

Major depressive episode, also called *major depression*, is a mood disorder seen in children and adolescents. The present system of psychiatric classification does not distinguish between adult and childhood depression, except to note a slightly different clinical picture. A mood characterized by sadness, feeling low, or hopelessness must be present for at least 2 weeks, or there must be a loss of pleasure or interest in usual activities if a diagnosis of major depression is to be made. Other criteria include impaired sleep, impaired appetite, increased or decreased restlessness, decreased ability to concentrate, and recurrent thoughts of death or suicide. If hallucinations or delusions are present, their content must be consistent with the child's mood—for example, a voice that criticizes the child for wrongdoing. Separation anxiety, with school refusal and fear that the parents may die, may be a symptom of depression in school-aged children. There is still controversy about exactly what constitutes the clinical symptoms of depression at different stages of childhood. This controversy will be resolved only when follow-up and family studies carefully define the natural history of these symptoms.

If depressive mood alternates with manic mood, *bipolar disorder* is considered. This disorder is not as common as the depressive disorders, and it is not often diagnosed in children and adolescents. Manic symptoms include elevated or irritable mood that is present for at least 1 week and that is accompanied by other symptoms, such as increased activity, overtalkativeness, distractibility, and poor judgment. Temper tantrums, anger, and aggressiveness are other reported symptoms of childhood manic disorder. Substance abuse is a common complication of manic disorder. Because certain manic symptoms are shared with conduct disorder and attention-deficit hyperactivity disorder, it is sometimes difficult to distinguish among these disorders. The presence of a bipolar disorder in other family members is important supportive evidence in making this diagnosis.

Children may also have a chronic depressive disorder called *dysthymia*. The symptoms are similar to those of major depression but hallucinations and delusions are not present. Social interaction with peers and adults and school performance frequently are impaired to a mild or moderate degree.

Childhood mood disorders may be treated effectively by a variety of individual and group therapies, including psychotherapy, behavior therapy, cognitive therapy, and family therapy. Medication may be given in combination with one of the above forms of therapy. The individual or group therapy helps the child and family to better understand their problems and to develop effective strategies to lessen the child's symptoms. The tricyclic antidepressants, most commonly imipramine, are the medications used in the treatment of childhood depressive disorders. Lithium and carbamazepine are used in the treatment of bipolar disorders. Whichever form of therapy is used, it is important to follow the course of certain symptoms, such as impaired appetite, difficulty in concentrating, and restless sleep, to monitor the child's progress. If medication is used, it is important to check for side effects at regular intervals. (See Chapter 4 for a detailed discussion of the medical treatment of these mood disorders.)

Organic Personality Syndrome

Organic mental syndromes refer to a group of behavioral or psychological abnormalities that are associated with temporary or permanent impairment of brain functioning. These disorders, among them delirium, the intoxications, and the withdrawals, are frequently seen in children.

Organic personality syndrome is one of the organic mental syndromes. This disorder is characterized by a persistent disturbance in the child's personality or behavior, and includes symptoms of mood fluctuation, poor impulse control, marked apathy and indifference, and suspiciousness or paranoid thinking. The specific clinical pattern of organic personality syndrome varies according to the nature and location of the brain impairment. Several clinical patterns have been described in childhood and adolescence. Two of these patterns are discussed here.

The first clinical pattern seen in children with organic personality syndrome is one of behavioral disinhibition. This lack of behavioral restraint can be seen as a consequence of severe closed head injury that involves the frontal lobes of the brain. Symptoms include inappropriate familiarity with strangers, overtalkativeness, messiness, use of obscenities, inappropriate sexual behavior, and lack of motivation. This clinical pattern bears some similarities to the syndrome described in adults following penetrating injuries to the frontal lobes. Symptoms of "frontal lobe syndrome" include (1) euphoria, (2) lack of judgment, reliability, or foresight, (3) disinhibition, (4) facile or childish behavior, and (5) apathy or loss of drive (Lishman, 1968). The following case history describes an adolescent who developed behavioral disinhibition during recovery from closed head injury.

Sixteen-year-old Andy suffered closed head injury in a fall from his bicycle. Cerebral and brainstem contusions and a right subdural hematoma were diagnosed. The patient was treated in intensive care and remained comatose for 4 weeks. Six months after his injury, Andy demonstrated long- and short-term memory deficits, together with significant receptive and expressive language deficits. He made frequent, rapid, very concrete associations. By 1 year after his injury, Andy's cognitive ability had gradually improved into the normal range.

Andy had a fairly good social adjustment before his injury. He returned to a small structured classroom at his high school, where he had been an eleventh grade student in a vocational placement. He was overtalkative, and his conversation frequently wandered from the topic. Furthermore, he was inappropriately friendly with classmates, and his humor was immature and sexually suggestive. Both his insight and his judgment were poor. Andy had been mildly overweight before his injury, but his eating increased greatly after his injury, and he gained 105 pounds in 1 year. Andy was manipulated and provoked by classmates, and he lost most of his former friends.

Andy's sexually disinhibited and mildly disruptive classroom behavior was troublesome to his teachers. The rehabilitation psychologist worked with the teaching staff to set up and help implement a behavior management program that targeted the following behaviors: inappropriate jokes, argumentativeness, and distraction of other students. This program was helpful in enabling Andy to graduate on schedule with his class (Gerring, 1985).

Andy's case demonstrates the first clinical pattern seen in children with organic personality syndrome: behavioral disinhibition.

The second clinical pattern includes aggression as the prominent symptom. This pattern may be seen in patients with epilepsy, most frequently with complex partial seizures, also called temporal lobe epilepsy. The aggression is sudden, immature, and inexplicable. It may occur as a feature of the seizure, but more commonly it appears between seizures. Other symptoms associated with this clinical pattern include impulsiveness, suspiciousness, overtalkativeness, and moodiness. The following case history describes an epileptic child who was suspended from school after assaulting a classmate.

Susan was a 12-year-old seventh grade student with a partial complex seizure disorder that was diagnosed at age 7 years. A CT scan showed a cyst in the right temporal lobe, and an EEG showed seizure activity involving both temporal lobes. Susan's seizures were well controlled with carbamazepine (Tegretol). She had a 4-year history of aggressive school behavior. Her grandmother complained of misbehaviors at home, including argumentativeness, disobedience, being suspicious, and talking too much. Just after the psychiatrist's first meeting with her, Susan physically attacked a classmate and was suspended from school. After the incident, she stated that the classmate had teased her about being fat. She said, "Just a few of the kids tease me, and the teachers don't handle it. But I don't sit and let the kids hit on me. If I sit there and let them hit on me, I'd have bruises on me." During the evaluation sessions, Susan was calm and superficially pleasant until anxiety-provoking material was raised or until her requests were not granted. Then she quickly became irritable, and, unless reassured, her irritability progressed to a state of anger.

Susan's behavior showed similarities to behavior seen in conduct disorder, solitary aggressive type. The psychiatrist searched for alternative or accompanying diagnoses, however, and noted the temporal lobe abnormality and the partial complex seizure disorder. This neurological history was important in leading to the diagnosis of organic personality syndrome. The medication used to treat Susan's seizure disorder, carbamazepine, has been beneficial in the treatment of aggressive behavior in many patients. In Susan's case, however, this medication was not beneficial. As her family was unable to manage her behavior, Susan was placed in a residential school in a program for brain damaged youngsters. Here a successful therapeutic program combined behavioral, psychosocial, and drug treatments.

Pervasive Developmental Disorders

Many terms have been used to describe children who have developmental disorders with severe behavioral and emotional symptoms. Some of these terms are listed in Table 2-2. They reflect a variety of theoretical views about the causation and treatment of these severe childhood disorders. Some of these children appear so disturbed behaviorally or emotionally that observers have described them as being out of touch with reality or psychotic, using terms such as childhood schizophrenia and symbiotic psychosis.

The DSM III-R classification system represents an attempt to standardize terminology and to take into account the social interactive, communicative, and behavioral deficits that are components of these developmental disorders. The disorders are defined in DSM III-R by clinical symptoms only; there is no reference to causation. The

TABLE 2-2.
Diagnostic Terms That Have Been Replaced by *Pervasive Developmental Disorders* and *Schizophrenic Disorder*

Atypical personality development	Infantile psychosis
Autistic psychopathy	Regressed ego state
Child schizophrenia	Schizophrenia, childhood type
Early childhood psychosis	Schizophrenic reaction, childhood type
Infantile autism	Symbiotic psychosis

implication of psychosis has been eliminated because it is difficult to judge a loss of contact with reality in a child whose social interaction, language, and behavior are severely impaired. Furthermore, DSM III-R's use of clear nonpsychiatric language to describe the symptoms of pervasive developmental disorders is helpful to the nonpsychiatric specialists who are involved with the treatment of these children. As more professionals adopt the present psychiatric classification system, greater amounts of shared information will be available to facilitate the understanding of these disorders.

There are two pervasive developmental disorders: *autistic disorder* and *pervasive developmental disorder, not otherwise specified*. All patients with these disorders demonstrate severe disturbances of the psychological functions involved in the development of social interaction and language. Autistic disorder has a prevalence of from 2 to 4 per 10,000 children and is about three times more common in boys than in girls. Most autistic children have an IQ in the retarded range. There is an increased incidence in siblings and in the presence of certain diseases such as maternal rubella, encephalitis, fragile X syndrome, and tuberous sclerosis. Autistic disorder is characterized by very poor social responsiveness, severe language deficits, and abnormal speech, if speech develops. Autistic behaviors include poor eye contact, an insistence on doing things the same way, under- or over-sensitivity to sensory stimuli, and stereotyped body movements. Some autistic children develop good language skills and improve in their social functioning as they grow older. Although they may have persistent social awkwardness and impaired communication, they manage to obtain some degree of independence. (See Chapter 7 for a more detailed discussion of autistic disorder and its treatment.)

There are many disturbed children and adolescents who meet some, but not all, of the diagnostic criteria for autistic disorder. These children can be given the diagnosis of pervasive developmental disorder, not otherwise specified. Other groups of children, such as children with severe language deficits and impaired social skills, still lie outside the present classification and are not given either diagnosis.

When disturbed children hallucinate or are delusional, the adult diagnosis of schizophrenic disorder is considered. Adult criteria include illness lasting at least 6 months, deterioration from a previous level of functioning, markedly illogical thinking, and specific types of hallucinations and delusions. Although the adult form of schizophrenia has been diagnosed in children as young as 5 years old, the disorder is rare in children younger than 7 years old. The prevalence rate of schizophrenic disorder in childhood is estimated to be far less than the rate of autistic disorder (Tanguay and Cantor, 1986).

The comprehensive treatment of these severe childhood disturbances includes educational, psychosocial, and medical methods. Educational methods used with severely emotionally handicapped children are discussed in Chapter 7. Although many medications have been used to treat children with pervasive developmental disorders, neuroleptics such as haloperidol (Haldol) and trifluoperazine (Stelazine) appear to be most beneficial. These medications work best to reduce the hyperactivity or agitation sometimes associated with these disorders. Medications are less effective in reducing the apathy that is seen in some of these children, however (Campbell, 1985). Although medical treatment may not have a direct beneficial effect on learning or social interaction, it may help to eliminate troublesome symptoms that prevent the development of adaptive social and learning skills. By modifying the child's interaction with the environment, these medications may facilitate the success of concurrently used educational and psychosocial treatment methods.

Sleep Disorders

Disorders of sleep are divided into two groups. The first group consists of disorders in the amount, quality, and timing of sleep. This group includes insomnia (difficulty in falling asleep) and hypersomnia (excessive sleepiness when awake). The second group of sleep disorders consists of events that occur during sleep or at the threshold between sleep and wakefulness. This group includes nightmares, sleep terrors, and sleepwalking. These disorders commonly begin in childhood.

Emotional influences may play a major or minor role in sleep disorders. For example, a child with insomnia may be anxious, fearful, or depressed. If a sleep disorder has a physical cause, it may be initiated or maintained by emotional factors. For example, sleepwalking occurs in certain children during the nonrapid eye movement stage of sleep, and these children have no consistently associated mental disorders. Their sleepwalking episodes are more likely to occur if they are fatigued, have experienced recent stress, or have taken a sedative or hypnotic before going to bed.

Stereotypy/Habit Disorder

Stereotypy/habit disorder describes intentional, repetitive, nonfunctional behaviors that cause physical injury to the child or markedly interfere with his or her normal activities. Stereotypic behaviors are frequently seen in children who are retarded or autistic but are occasionally seen in normal children as well. Body-rocking and head-banging may occasionally be troublesome symptoms in normal children and may lead parents to inquire whether their children are normal or whether the head-banging will lead to brain damage. Nose-picking, nail-biting, and mouthing of objects are other behaviors that concern parents. These behaviors tend to lessen as the child ages, although body-rocking as an aid to sleep may persist into adolescence.

Stereotypy may be a prominent feature of retarded children's behavior, sometimes occupying several hours each day. These children repeat sequences of individual movements—for example, a limp-wristed, rapid shaking of both hands or a short loud burst of clapping. Children may look at their fingers, shake them and then flap them. One theory is that these movements help the child maintain an optimal level of stimulation; they are, therefore, sometimes referred to as self-stimulatory behaviors.

The frequency of these movements depends on circumstances in the environment. In general, these movements occur less often when the child is actively involved in closely supervised activities. On the other hand, these abnormal behaviors increase when socially appropriate behavior is not fostered and supervision is minimal.

Stereotypic behaviors are undesirable because they prevent cognitive and social growth. The time spent in hand-flapping is unavailable for learning and practicing new cognitive skills. Children with stereotypic behaviors also have fewer positive interactions with adults. Adults tend either to ignore the children when they are engaged in these movements or to respond to the movements in a negative way (Baumeister, MacLean, Kelly, and Kasari, 1980).

SUMMARY

Handicapped youngsters frequently develop psychiatric symptoms and disorders. These symptoms and disorders may constitute an additional handicap. When the symptoms become maladaptive, the child is referred for psychiatric evaluation. In this chapter the DSM III-R system of classification of mental disorders was described first. This was followed by a description of the psychiatric evaluation and the symptoms and disorders seen most commonly in handicapped children and adolescents.

When a psychiatrist has evaluated a child and diagnosed a mental disorder, he or she presents the diagnosis and treatment alternatives to those therapists involved with the youngster. The psychiatric treatment that is chosen depends on the disorder, the child's underlying handicap, the availability of the desired treatment, and the fit of the chosen psychiatric therapy with the other therapies the child is already receiving.

REFERENCES

Achenbach, T.M. (1980). DSM III in light of empirical research on the classification of child psychopathology. *Journal of the American Academy of Child Psychiatry, 19,* 395–412.

American Psychiatric Association. (1980). *Diagnostic and statistical manual of mental disorders* (3rd ed.). Washington, DC: Author.

American Psychiatric Association. (1987). *Diagnostic and statistical manual of mental disorders* (3rd ed.—revised). Washington, DC: Author.

Anderson, J.C., Williams, S., McGee, R., and Silva, P.A. (1987). DSM III disorders in preadolescent children. *Archives of General Psychiatry, 44,* 69–76.

Association for Advancement of Behavior Therapy Task Force Report. (1982). The treatment of self-injurious behavior. *Behavior Therapy, 13,* 529–554.

Baumeister, A.A., MacLean, W.E., Jr., Kelly, J., and Kasari, C. (1980). Observational studies of retarded children with multiple stereotyped movements. *Journal of Abnormal Child Psychology, 8,* 501–521.

Brown, G., and Harris, T. (1978). *Social origins of depression: The study of psychiatric disorder in women.* London: Tavistock.

Burke, P., Del Beccaro, M., McCauley, E., and Clark, C. (1985). Hallucinations in children. *Journal of the American Academy of Child Psychiatry, 24,* 71–75.

Campbell, M. (1985). Schizophrenic disorders and pervasive developmental disorders/infantile autism. In J. M. Wiener (Ed.), *Diagnosis and psychopharmacology of childhood and adolescent disorders* (pp. 114–150). New York: John Wiley and Sons.

Cantwell, D.P. (1980). The diagnostic process and diagnostic classification in child psychiatry. DSM III: Introduction. *Journal of the American Academy of Child Psychiatry, 19,* 345–355.

Conners, C.K. (1969). A teacher rating scale for use in drug studies with children. *American Journal of Psychiatry, 126,* 884–888.

Edelbrock, C., and Achenbach, T. (1984). The teacher version of the child behavior profile: 1. Boys aged 6–11. *Journal of Consulting and Clinical Psychology, 52,* 207–217.

Ferber, R. (1985). *Solve your child's sleep problems.* New York: Simon and Schuster, Inc.

Flament, M.F., Rapoport, J.L., Berg, C.J., Sceery, W., Kitts, C., Mellstrom, B., and Linnoila, M. (1985). Clomipramine treatment of childhood obsessive compulsive disorder: A double-blind controlled study. *Archives of General Psychiatry, 42,* 977–983.

Fraiberg, S. (1950). On the sleep disturbances of early childhood. *The Psychoanalytic Study of the Child, 5,* 285–309.

Freud, A. (1972). The concept of developmental lines. In S.I. Harrison and J.F. McDermott (Eds.), *Childhood psychopathology* (pp. 133–156). New York: International Universities Press, Inc.

Gardner, R.A. (1979). *The objective diagnosis of minimal brain dysfunction.* Cresskill, New Jersey: Creative Therapeutics.

Gerring, J.P. (1985). The diagnosis, treatment, and rehabilitation of severe closed head injury. In A.N. O'Quinn (Ed.), *Management of chronic disorders of childhood* (pp. 179–224). Boston: G.K. Hall Medical Publishers.

Gittelman, R. (1980). The role of psychological tests for differential diagnosis in child psychiatry. *Journal of the American Academy of Child Psychiatry, 19,* 413–438.

Gittelman-Klein, R., and Klein, D.F. (1971). Controlled imipramine treatment of school phobia. *Archives of General Psychiatry, 25,* 204–207.

Graham, P., and Rutter, M. (1970). Selection of children with psychiatric disorder. In M. Rutter, J. Tizard, and K. Whitmore (Eds.), *Education, health and behavior* (pp. 147–177). New York: John Wiley and Sons.

Horowitz, M.J. (1976). *Stress-response syndromes.* New York: Jason Aronson, Inc.

Lewis, D.O. (1985). Child delinquents who later commit murder have identifiable traits, study suggests. *Psychiatric News,* June 21, pp. 32–34.

Lishman, W.A. (1968). Brain damage in relation to psychiatric disability after head injury. *British Journal of Psychiatry, 114,* 373–410.

Loeber, R., and Dishion, T. (1983). Early predictors of male delinquency: A review. *Psychological Bulletin, 94,* 68–99.

Looker, A., and Conners, C.K. (1970). Diphenylhydantoin in children with severe temper tantrums. *Archives of General Psychiatry, 23,* 80–89.

McManus, M., Alessi, N., Grapentine, W.L., and Brickman, A. (1984). Psychiatric disturbance in serious delinquents. *Journal of the American Academy of Child Psychiatry, 23,* 602–615.

Millichamp, J.G., Aymat, F., Sturgis, L.H., Larsen, K.W., and Egan, R.A. (1968). Hyperkinetic behavior and learning disorders: II. Battery of neuropsychological tests in controlled trial of methylphenidate. *American Journal of the Diseases of Childhood, 116,* 235–244.

O'Donnell, D.J. (1985). Conduct disorders. In J.M. Wiener (Ed.), *Diagnosis and psychopharmacology of childhood and adolescent disorders* (pp. 249–287). New York: John Wiley and Sons.

Pfeffer, C.R., Zuckerman, S., Plutchik, R., and Mizruhi, M. (1984). Suicidal behavior in normal school children: A comparison with child psychiatric inpatients. *Journal of the American Academy of Child Psychiatry, 23,* 416–423.

Puig-Antich, J. (1982a). Major depression and conduct disorder in prepuberty. *Journal of the American Academy of Child Psychiatry, 21,* 118–128.

Puig-Antich, J. (1982b). The use of RDC criteria for major depressive disorder in children and adolescents. *Journal of the American Academy of Child Psychiatry, 21,* 291–293.

Shaywitz, S.E., and Shaywitz, B.A. (1984). Evaluation and treatment of children with attention deficit disorders. *Pediatrics in Review, 6,* 99–109.

Spitzer, R.L., and Cantwell, D.P. (1980). The DSM III classification of the psychiatric disorders of infancy, childhood, and adolescents. *Journal of the American Academy of Child Psychiatry, 19,* 356–370.

Tanguay, P.E., and Cantor, S.L. (1986). Schizophrenia in children. Introduction. *Journal of the American Academy of Child Psychiatry, 25,* 591–594.

Thomas, A., and Chess, S. (1984). Genesis and evolution of behavioral disorders: From infancy to early adult life. *American Journal of Psychiatry, 141,* 1–9.

Weinberg, W.A., and Brumback, R.A. (1976). Mania in childhood: Case studies and literature review. *American Journal of Diseases of Childhood, 130,* 380–385.

CHAPTER 3

BEHAVIORAL AND EMOTIONAL CONDITIONS OF HANDICAPPED ADOLESCENTS

Joan P. Gerring

Adolescence is the period between childhood and the adult years, which begins with the physicial transformation of puberty and ends with the attainment of psychological maturity. Adolescence in our culture is believed to culminate in financial and psychological independence, and thus it may not necessarily end with the teenage years. Rather, prolonged dependency on parents is common in our culture, and the result is often an adolescent period extending into the middle 20s and beyond.

Although adolescents must accomplish many difficult developmental tasks during this period of growth, it is, nonetheless, a stable and relatively peaceful time for most youngsters (Oldham, 1978). However, some 18 to 20 percent of adolescents experience emotional disturbance and may exhibit psychiatric symptoms (Kashani et al., 1987; Offer, 1987). If a handicap is present, an adolescent is more vulnerable for the development of disturbances and symptom formation.

In this chapter the developmental tasks of adolescence as they apply to the handicapped population are discussed. Case studies and discussion of the common behavioral and emotional conditions of handicapped adolescents are then presented. Adolescent pregnancy will be discussed as a behavioral condition that is especially stressful in handicapped youth. (See also Chapter 8 for a discussion of the tasks and needs of families with handicapped adolescents.)

THE HANDICAPPED CHILD JUST BEFORE ADOLESCENCE

Most children enter adolescence more or less equipped to handle the developmental tasks of this stage. Depending on their abilities, motivations, and environments, they have achieved some degree of mastery in physical, cognitive, social, and emotional areas. They are usually able to function independently to some degree and have achieved some control over bodily functions and internal impulses. They have also developed a set of coping strategies to help them deal with novel or stressful events.

Handicapped children have lived with additional psychological and psychosocial stresses. These stresses vary with the nature of the handicap and its mode of onset, as noted in Chapter 1. A child with a highly visible orthopedic deformity will experience different stresses than a child with normal appearance who is mentally retarded. From the onset of the handicap, the child's and family's perception of it affects the child's psychological functioning, and even the mislabeling of a normal child as handicapped can result in the child's and family's acting as if the child were disabled. Furthermore, the longer a handicap or a suspected handicap has been present, the greater the likelihood that it will have a lasting effect on the child's personality functioning.

Handicaps imply dependency. The more severe the handicap, the greater the dependency the child will have on parents or caregivers. Nonhandicapped children have often attained some degree of independence and are likely to view with confidence their increasing independence from their parents. Although dependent handicapped children may desire increasing independence, they often find it difficult to imagine as a realistic goal. Those handicapped children who are less dependent may wish for eventual complete independence, but they are unsure whether they will be able to attain it.

All handicapped children develop coping strategies in response to their handicap and dependency. Some become passive and resigned to their dependent state and appear unmotivated to change their condition. Some of these children become masochistic, with an apparent need for the pity of others. Other children become angry about their dependent conditions and project their anger onto their caregivers. This hostile response to their dependent state probably is common in severely handicapped children who can see no future lessening of their dependency. Still other handicapped children develop the behavioral or emotional symptoms discussed in Chapters 2 and 4, such as aggression, anxiety, and depression.

As stated in Chapter 1, the incidence of behavioral and emotional disorders is high in children with handicaps. Those physically and/or mentally handicapped children who have developed emotional and behavioral problems as well enter adolescence with the second handicap of psychiatric disorder. This will make accomplishing the tasks of adolescence even more difficult. For example, a child with a learning disability and resultant lowered self-esteem will enter adolescence with two handicaps (learning disability and lowered self-esteem). Another child with attention-deficit hyperactivity disorder (ADHD) who develops an aggressive conduct disorder also enters adolescence with two disorders. This compounding of problems obviously places these teenagers at a disadvantage as they begin to work on the developmental tasks of adolescence.

There are, of course, handicapped children who have traversed childhood in an adaptive fashion. These children may have cognitive, emotional, or motor strengths that compensate for their areas of deficit. They may also have had a supportive family, which enabled them to negotiate their stressful circumstances successfully. At the end of childhood they are functioning successfully in home, school, and leisure activities. Despite their handicaps, they have achieved some degree of mastery over themselves and their environment and have adequate self-esteem. When discussing the handicapped adolescent, it is important to distinguish at the outset between those children who have had troubled childhoods and those children whose childhoods were calmer and relatively normal.

THE DEVELOPMENTAL TASKS OF ADOLESCENCE

The developmental tasks of adolescence are the same for all youngsters, normal and handicapped. These tasks include adjustment to a changing body image, progression toward independence from the family, creation of a mature identity, formation of realistic goals, development of the capacity to defer gratification, and the formation of caring and intimate relationships (Grob, 1986). A youngster's handicap may well affect the accomplishment of these tasks.

Adjustment to a Changing Body Image

The accommodation to a changing body image will be influenced by whether or not a part of the body is handicapped. Physical development causes increased awareness of one's body and emphasizes to a physically handicapped youth that his or her body is not whole and entire. Physical and sexual development in a youth with a mental handicap also raises questions about the eventual level of social and sexual functioning.

There is additional concern for mentally handicapped adolescent girls. Depending on the severity of their retardation, these girls will vary in their ability to handle their menses. Of greater concern, however, is protecting them from undesired sexual advances and unwanted pregnancy. The concern for adolescent retarded males is different; it is often their inappropriate and disinhibited behavior that is a worry to their parents.

Parents are less likely to attempt total care of an adolescent with a severe handicap than they are the total care of a younger child with a similar handicap. Such severe handicaps include quadriplegia, ventilator dependency, and vegetative state (a condition of behavioral unresponsiveness). Apparently caring for a completely dependent younger child is more bearable to families than caring for a completely dependent adolescent or young adult. The physical burden of caring for the heavier, helpless body of an adolescent no doubt plays a role.

It is often difficult for parents to accommodate to the physical and sexual development of their handicapped child. As their normal children get older, their growth and increased sexual maturity remind parents that these children will become more independent. As handicapped children mature, however, their parents are unsure of the degree of independence that their child will attain.

Progression Toward Independence from the Family

Teenagers normally separate from their parents and become more independent, although financial independence and marriage may not come until later. Both adolescents and their families view the years from 13 to 20 as a time of gradual loosening of the strong psychological bonds of childhood.

It is different, however, when the child is handicapped. There is a wide spectrum of handicapping conditions, varying in duration and severity from a transitory medical illness, such as acute rheumatic fever, to remediable learning disabilities to severe permanent conditions, such as quadriplegia and ventilator dependency. When a handicap is temporary or does not result in permanent incapacity, there is usually little concern about the eventual attainment of independence. In cases in which the handicaps are more severe and long-lasting, the issue of eventual independence becomes important to both teenagers and their parents. If adolescents believe that their handicaps prevent progress, their self-esteem may lessen. Their uncertainty and discouragement about eventual self-sufficiency may also lead to the development of psychiatric symptoms, such as anxiety or depression.

It is possible for severely handicapped adolescents to attain some degree of separateness from their families. An adaptive teenager with a supportive family can learn many personal skills and take up activities, such as sports or music, that encourage functioning outside the family.

Even within the confines of severe dependency, parents can treat the handicapped adolescent as a mature person, and he or she can respond in a mature manner.

As parents perceive that their handicapped child will remain dependent, they must consider future care. Sometimes parents turn to siblings or other relatives to assume responsibility for care when they are no longer able to perform these tasks. At times parents may be angry that there will be no time when they will be free of child care responsibilities. The more severe the handicap, the higher the possibility that institutional care will be considered. If the child enters an institution, the physical burden on the parents may decrease, but their psychological burden, which often includes guilt, may remain or even increase.

Creation of a Mature Identity

A person's identity is formed by the interaction of many components—cognitive, psychological, physical, sexual, and motor. It is also formed through identifications with parents, idealized adults, and peers. When adolescents are handicapped in one of the aforementioned areas or when their interactions with others are impaired, their eventual perceptions of themselves and their place in the world will be affected.

The effect of handicap on a child's identity formation depends on how severe the handicap is and how it is perceived. This can be seen in two examples. In the first, a 4-year-old girl's heart murmur was misdiagnosed as serious heart disease. As a result, the child was perceived as being chronically ill and was severely restricted in physical activities. The child, her family, and her community viewed her as ill and accepted these restrictions. Each choice that the child or family made was governed by the presumption of illness, and cardiac disease (albeit imagined) became part of the child's self-image.

A second example of the effect of handicap on identity formation concerns a child with a noticeable physical handicap who compensated in other areas. Lussier (1960) described a 13-year-old boy with noticeably malformed arms who did not perceive himself as handicapped. As a teenager, he compensated for the lack of normal arms by becoming involved in activities in which good physical functioning was necessary. Despite initial fears that others had for his safety, the teenager became a good diver. He played the trumpet with some modification and developed his interest to the extent that he wished to form his own band. His cognitive, sexual, and social development proceeded in a fairly uneventful and normal manner. The adolescent course of this remarkable youth, whether attributed to temperament, motivation, abilities, coping strategies, or environmental circumstances, provides an optimistic picture of the potential for mature identity formation under circumstances of severe handicap.

Formation of Realistic Goals

The ability to formulate realistic goals is an extension of the process of identity formation. Once teenagers have a stable notion of who they are, they can plan for the future. Although adolescents vary widely in their ability to form goals for themselves, and at first these goals may be hazy and unrealistic, they generally become clearer as the adolescent matures. Handicapped adolescents often have more difficulty in setting goals than do their nonhandicapped peers.

There are, however, well-known examples of individuals who have overcome severe handicaps to excel in physical or mental endeavors. The teenaged boy described earlier is such a person. Other examples include a teenager with a severe foot deformity who was motivated to condition himself and eventually became an excellent runner. Another teenager with a similar handicap was motivated to excel in mathematics, an academic pursuit unrelated to the physical handicap. Sometimes teenagers receive encouragement from their parents, but at other times the motivation is all their own.

Many handicapped youths falter in their abilities to set up realistic goals. Depending on their degrees of dependency, they may rely on their families to set up their goals for the future. Although they may not be content with their families' decisions, they view these decisions as the only reasonable alternatives. They may believe that if financial and social independence are not to be attainable goals, they may as well passively accept the direction provided by the family. Again this resolution may work well in some cases but leads to chronic anger in others. These angry adolescents may be in frequent conflict with their caregivers.

Some handicapped adolescents and their families are confused about the possibility of attaining certain goals. The adolescents wonder if a vocational choice is inappropriate because it is beyond their abilities or if they will be comfortable with a certain lifestyle. Parents' and adolescents' uncertainties can stem from incomplete information or from the failure to understand what they've been told. If the clinical course and prognosis of their handicap is not yet completely understood by professionals, as is the case with many handicaps such as learning disabilities and head injuries, this lack of knowledge must be transmitted constructively to parents. Even when professionals believe they have adequately informed handicapped adolescents and their families, however, gaps in understanding may occur if care is not consistent or there is no primary caregiver or case manager. Especially in adolescence, handicapped youths may need professional help to understand what is happening to them and to help them make reasonable decisions about the future.

Goals of adolescence include, as already stated, social and financial independence. This most often is viewed as getting married and establishing one's own household. Currently, however, other lifestyles—living alone, living with another adult without marriage, and living in small or large organized groups—are options. A handicapped person who is unable to live alone may elect to live in a supervised group home in the community where he or she will be able to have privacy and some degree of responsibility. For example, group homes have been established for youths with severe retardation, for youths with pervasive developmental disorders, and for youths with other severe emotional disturbances. The goals for independent functioning and the type of supervision for these three categories of handicapped young people are very different.

Because of the difficulties of setting vocational goals, handicapped adolescents often need assistance in making vocational decisions. Guidance should take place informally during the early teenage years and in a more formal fashion during the middle teenage years. Educators should inform youngsters about possible vocations and bring in people employed in these vocations to speak to students about them. Field trips to employment areas are also helpful. When adolescents are capable and interested, assignment can be made to specialized high schools where time is divided between academic and vocational subjects. Vocational guidance is more difficult, however, for students with severe physical and mental incapacities. Vocational opportunities are very limited and often must be specially created.

State departments of vocational rehabilitation work with special educators to assess students' potentials and provide necessary training to integrate handicapped youths into suitable employment. Because the school system is responsible for handicapped youngsters until the age of 21 years, special education now assumes a responsibility for vocational guidance. In optimal circumstances, there will be a period of overlap when the school and the vocational rehabilitation system work together in vocational guidance and placement.

Capacity to Defer Gratification

The capacity to make good choices and to defer gratification develops gradually during childhood. The capacity to manage stressful events is a related goal. Through trial and error, children learn to choose and to wait. Cognitive abilities play an important role in being able

to develop and consider a range of alternatives. Components of temperament, such as the level of sensory threshold and degree of persistence,
may also influence a child's ability to think things out before acting.
A persistent child with a high sensory threshold is more likely to consider alternatives than an impatient child who responds rapidly at a
lower level of stimulation.

In addition to intelligence level and temperament, the family
environment is important in the development of children's ability to
make good choices. Children tend to copy their parents' ability to
organize themselves, to consider worthwhile alternatives, to
thoughtfully choose the best alternative, and to learn from the outcome
of their decisions. Ideally parents should help their children make good
choices and help them manage their disappointments and other
stressful situations. Disorganized families with impulsive members,
however, are subject to multiple stresses and are often too burdened
to profit from lessons of past mistakes or to help their children make
good choices.

The special challenge of handicapped adolescents is to develop the
ability to handle the crises and stresses related to their handicaps. The
capacity of these youngsters and their families to adapt to the stress
of chronic handicap undoubtedly influences the outcome. In an
outcome study of young adults with severe head injuries, good family
support resulted in a higher percentage of patients who returned to
their homes and former jobs (Gilchrist and Wilkinson, 1979).

Capacity for Caring and Intimate Relationships

The capacity to develop intimate, give-and-take friendships
develops during childhood and early adolescence, and as children grow
older they develop a characteristic style of relating to others. Initially,
a child learns from family members' interactions with one another,
although as time goes on, the outside environment plays an increasingly important role.

The formation in adolescence or early adulthood of an enduring
sexual relationship is more complicated than the formation of childhood
friendships. The capacity for a mature and lasting sexual relationship
implies a secure self-image and a mature identity along with the ability
to empathize and to compromise with others. This developmental task
is especially difficult in the presence of physical and mental handicap.

The capacity to relate to others in a mature fashion also implies
some degree of independent functioning. When dependency has been
prolonged or extreme, the dependent people remain in childlike positions of inequality. Even when they are motivated, they are often unable

to pursue give-and-take relationships. The natural desire for a satisfying sexual relationshp may not be fulfilled because of the severity of the handicap, or the desire may be discouraged by the family because they are concerned about the adolescent's ability to function in such a relationship. In the past, such fears about the sexual vulnerability of handicapped youth led to sterilization procedures that clearly were not indicated.

Social isolation is also a problem for many adolescents with moderate and severe handicaps. This isolation may develop despite an adequate social adjustment during childhood. Even when handicapped children have done well in regular elementary school classes, their entry into adolescence may signal new social difficulties. Chess and coworkers described a 13-year-old girl with profound deafness who had made a good academic and social adjustment during childhood (Chess, Fernandez, and Korn, 1980). Relationships with normal peers became increasingly stressful during adolescence, however. Her lip reading ability was no longer adequate to keep up with the rapid verbal communication of her peers, and her own speech became more difficult for her classmates to understand. Although some classmates remained sympathetic, others mocked and teased her. When such social isolation occurs, parents often consider transferring of their handicapped youngster to a special day school or a residential facility.

The sudden onset of handicap during adolescence may also lead to social isolation and decreased opportunities for socialization. Teenagers who have suffered a severe closed head injury may have permanent cognitive and personality deficits. Former friends and classmates see that the head injured youth is no longer the same person but, rather, someone slower, or disinhibited, or apathetic, or with obviously inappropriate responses. At first, former friends may try hard to maintain the friendship, but other interests and other people hold more attraction, and soon the visits decrease and then cease. Again, parents may feel powerless to secure socialization experiences that seem natural and not contrived. In such situations, church or community groups may be helpful in providing opportunities for handicapped youths to become involved in activity or social groups.

Adolescents with lesser degrees of handicap may also have difficulty in establishing caring and intimate relationships. Some adolescents with attention-deficit hyperactivity disorder (ADHD), a relatively minor handicap, have an impaired ability to socialize with peers. Symptoms of impulsivity and inattention may prevent these youngsters from working out problems in relationships. Rather, they interrupt and do not listen to what others say. Even the perception of handicap, as already stated, may result in an overprotective environment in which an adolescent may remain immature or passive for a prolonged period.

Coping with Sexuality and Pregnancy

The sexuality of the disabled is one of the most difficult aspects of handicap. Neither disabled adolescents nor their caregivers should be expected to deal with this difficult aspect of functioning totally on their own. Education and counseling of youngsters and their caregivers is necessary to discuss what is possible and practical. The school system is in a position to provide leadership in this process of psychosexual education for the handicapped. Although there is not yet a solid research foundation in this area, interested professionals have accumulated a considerable amount of useful clinical information. The following case history illustrates the complex and difficult problem that sexuality and pregnancy present for handicapped young adults and their caregivers.

Saralee was a well-adjusted, high functioning high school student whose sudden brain injury resulted in a new and incapacitating mental disorder. Her mental disorder was further complicated by two unplanned pregnancies 2 and 3 years after her injury.

Saralee was a 17-year-old adolescent who suffered severe traumatic brain injury as a pedestrian crossing the street on her way to school. She was a high school senior who had been involved in many school and church activities and planned to attend college. After she was injured, she remained in a coma for 19 days. As she recovered, her intelligence returned to a normal range, but her thinking was very disordered. Although her train of thought could be followed, she was overtalkative and could not stay on a topic of conversation. She became overly familiar with strangers. Her emotional reactions were unpredictable and often inappropriate to the occasion. One year after her injury Saralee was given the psychiatric diagnosis of organic personality disorder.

Saralee participated in a cognitive rehabilitation program for head injured adults and received encouragement and guidance from her entire family and from her social worker-therapist. Two years after her injury, she enrolled in a state university program for students with learning disabilities. She remained in college for several months, but she was unable to organize her time and pass her course work.

Saralee's disinhibited behavior caused concern to her family and her social worker. They gave her birth control advice, and she decided to take birth control pills. However, she became pregnant 2 years after her injury, supposedly while she was taking the pills. This pregnancy ended in a miscarriage at $2\frac{1}{2}$ months. A year later, Saralee became pregnant again and married the father before the baby's birth. The father's family helped Saralee care for the infant, who subsequently died of sudden infant death syndrome at 5 months of age. After the death, Saralee entered a bookkeeping training program run by the Maryland State Department of Vocational Rehabilitation. At present she is still in that program.

Pregnancy may be viewed as a handicapping condition in some school systems when it contributes to poor academic performance. Pregnancy is often stressful to the unmarried teenager, who is unprepared for the physical, mental, and social responsibility of parenting. In the case of Saralee, handicapped by a severe mental disorder, pregnancy and parenting constituted an extreme stress.

In launching a comprehensive teen health project, the American Medical Association has focused on teenage sexuality and pregnancy. According to the AMA, this is one of the five major factors contributing to increasing impairment of physical and mental health in United States teenagers (*American Medical News*, 1986, p. 4). A few statistics emphasize the urgent nature of the problem. The teenage pregnancy rate in this country is the second highest of all industrialized counties. Eighty percent of male teenagers and 70 percent of female teenagers in this country will have had intercourse by age 19 years (Alan Guttmacher Institute, 1985). Most teenagers wait at least 9 months after their first sexual encounter before they seek contraceptive advice, and 1.1 million of these teenagers become pregnant each year: that represents 11 percent of the 15- to 19-year-old population. Less than 20 percent of these pregnancies are conceived in marriage. About half end in childbirth, and half end in abortion. Many interacting factors—poverty, racism, urbanization, and the permissive sexual norms of the larger society—have contributed to the high incidence of teenage sex and pregnancy (Chilman, 1983).

Pregnancy prevention programs work to decrease the teenage pregnancy rate by reducing sexual activity and by preventing pregnancy in sexually active teens. Zabin and her colleagues designed and administered a model pregnancy prevention program at two inner city junior and two inner city senior high schools in Baltimore (Zabin, 1986). This program did not include handicapped students, but it may be instructive to those professionals who work with handicapped adolescents.

In the four schools in which Zabin worked, basic sex education programs already existed. In addition, these students favored contraception and opposed early pregnancy before the new prevention program began. The program combined education, counseling, and contraceptive services, both in the schools and in a special clinic close to the schools. This school-based approach stressed responsible sexual behavior, postponement of sexual intercourse, and open communication with parents. It also helped students place their sexual conduct in the context of personal goals and values. This program lasted for three academic years and involved 1700 male and female students. It was evaluated by self-administered questionnaires at four different times during the study.

This program achieved several notable results: (1) The pregnancy rates of these students decreased; (2) students' sexual and contraceptive knowledge increased; (3) students sought pregnancy prevention methods sooner after beginning sexual activity than they had previously; (4) the effects of the program were greater among younger than among older students; (5) junior high school boys, a difficult group to reach, used the services to the same extent as did the junior high school girls (Zabin et al, 1986).

There was little measurable change in the attitudes of these students during the time of the study, although it was believed that the program helped those students with positive attitudes toward pregnancy prevention translate their attitudes into action. That students who were exposed to the entire program postponed their sexual activity refutes the argument that providing knowledge and contraceptive services invites sexual activity.

Sexuality Counseling

There is no study comparable to Zabin's that focuses on handicapped students or students in special education. Handicapped adolescents, however, as they develop sexually, also have needs for education, counseling, and contraceptive services. Programs for handicapped adolescents will have to be modified according to the youngsters' types of handicap. The degree of eventual sexual independence possible for the involved youth will affect program planning decisions.

For example, sex education for a moderately retarded teenager may be a simple explanation of anatomy, menstruation, and intercourse. The youth may be counseled about interactions with those people that he or she finds sexually attractive. If retarded adolescents are capable of using contraceptives, they should be assisted in initial selection and use. Furthermore, because masturbation is an important means of sexual expression in retarded individuals, it should be discussed with youngsters. They should be counseled concerning its use so that it provides sexual satisfaction in a private rather than in a public environment (Gilchrist and Schinke, 1983). Adolescents with physical and sensory handicaps need other program modifications. Physical impediments to proper hygiene or sexual performance should be discussed along with solutions to these problems.

When a chronic handicap and a lengthy period of dependence are anticipated, the family's role in sex education and counseling is especially important. The greater the degree of handicap, the more likely it is that the adolescent will be dependent, isolated, and immature in his or her social interactions. Such a situation understandably makes parents apprehensive about sexual enlightenment and contraceptive services for their child. Adolescent sexuality programs designed for the handicapped must acknowledge this apprehension and work with families to establish reasonable goals.

MENTAL DISORDERS IN ADOLESCENCE

There is a high incidence of mental disorder in adolescents with physical and mental handicaps. The reasons for this were discussed in Chapter 1. The mental disorders of handicapped adolescents are the same as those of nonhandicapped adolescents, but certain disorders occur more frequently in populations with certain handicaps. For example, in 113 adolescents with developmental disabilities who were referred for psychiatric evaluation, the most frequent diagnosis was conduct disorder, seen in 38 percent of that population. Poor socialization and aggressive behavior were common in these retarded teenagers. The lower frequency of emotional disorders, such as anxiety, withdrawal, and depression, in moderately and severely retarded teenagers was attributed to these teenagers' lack of awareness about their condition (Myers, 1987).

This discussion of mental disorders in adolescence will begin by focusing on three behavioral and emotional conditions commonly seen in handicapped adolescents: attention-deficit hyperactivity disorder, conduct/antisocial disorder, and substance abuse. The case history used to illustrate these three conditions is that of an 18-year-old boy, Kevin, who suffered severe brain injury in a car accident. Traumatic brain injuries usually occur in adolescents who have a history of behavioral or emotional disorder, and these disorders often play a role in causing the accident. In the case of Kevin, behavioral disorder preceded his injury and complicated his recovery.

Kevin was an 18-year-old boy who suffered severe head injury as a passenger in a speeding automobile. Both Kevin and the driver were intoxicated, and illegal drugs were found in the car. Kevin remained comatose for 5 days. As he emerged from coma, his behavior toward the staff became verbally and physically aggressive. For example, if Kevin's activities were restricted, he would hit his caregiver or throw a nearby object across the room. The patient was transferred to a rehabilitation hospital, where, within several days, his motor and cognitive abilities approached a normal level, although recent memory deficits persisted. Behavioral methods and major tranquilizers were used to control Kevin's aggressive behavior, but his repeated attempts to leave the hospital led to his transfer to a psychiatric unit for further treatment.

Kevin was the second of four sons. A tracheoesophageal fistula, a severe congenital abnormality, was diagnosed 36 hours after birth. Corrective surgery was performed, but Kevin had frequent hospitalizations for respiratory infections until he was 7 years old. At age 5 years, he was hospitalized for head injury and a brief period of unconsciousness. When he was 8 years old, he was given dextroamphetamine (Dexedrine) for symptoms of hyperactivity, inattention, and impulsivity. Improvement occurred in these symptoms, but the family chose not to continue medication. Although school performance was poor and Kevin was retained in the fourth grade, he was never evaluated for the presence of learning disabilities. At age 9 years, migraine headaches were diagnosed. Somewhat immature speech and a mild lisp were noted at that time.

As Kevin's schooling progressed, he was frequently truant and became increasingly aggressive in the classroom. At the time of the car accident, Kevin had been on probation three times for aggressive delinquent acts, including tire slashing. He was drunk on at least one of these occasions. It is of interest that both Kevin's father and his older brother had had past episodes of drunken driving and severe head trauma.

Kevin was, thus, an adolescent who had had a number of childhood problems, including repair and lengthy rehabilitation of a major congenital abnormality, attention-deficit hyperactivity disorder (ADHD), and a speech disorder. School performance was poor. Aggressive behavior and truancy had appeared in early adolescence, and by age 18 years, at the time of the accident, Kevin had become involved with delinquent behavior and substance abuse. The accident resulted in a persistent memory deficit and in an exacerbation of his previously aggressive behavior.

Although Kevin had multiple childhood problems that contributed to his difficult adolescence, his history is not unusual. The sequence of events in Kevin's case is consistent with the natural history of ADHD now being clarified by clinical research studies. Kevin's disorders— ADHD, conduct/antisocial disorder, and substance abuse—all present in this handicapped patient, are three psychiatric disorders commonly seen in adolescents.

Attention-Deficit Hyperactivity Disorder

The symptoms of ADHD continue into adolescence in the majority of affected children. During adolescence, the behavior of many of these children normalizes. Full symptoms of ADHD were still present in 35 percent of one study's 18-year-old population, however (Gittelman, Mannuzza, Shenker, and Bonagura, 1985). Poor academic performance and impaired social skills continued to be disabling problems for these adolescents. Teenagers who retained symptoms of ADHD were, like Kevin, at high risk for the development of conduct/antisocial disorder and delinquent behavior: 48 percent of the adolescents in Gittelman and colleagues' study who continued to have ADHD also had conduct disorders. Family factors and aggressive behavior in early childhood also predict antisocial behavior in hyperactive adolescents (Weiss, 1983). In one controlled study of adolescent boys with ADHD, there was a strong relationship between ADHD and later arrest for delinquent behaviors (Satterfield, Hoppe, and Schell, 1982).

Two important aspects of the relationship between ADHD and substance abuse must be considered. The first aspect concerns the effect of psychostimulant medication on adolescents with ADHD. It was earlier thought that the stimulant properties of dextroamphetamine amd methylphenidate would appear during adolescence and that the beneficial effects of these drugs on hyperactivity, inattention, and impulsivity would no longer occur. There is now evidence, however, that the psychostimulants continue to exert a beneficial effect on ADHD symptoms in young adults (Gittelman-Klein, 1987).

A second consideration is whether psychostimulant usage in adolescence leads to substance abuse. In Gittelman and colleagues' study (1985), most of the ADHD adolescents who abused substances had a prior history of conduct or antisocial disorder, and the frequency of conduct or antisocial disorder was high in adolescents in whom ADHD symptoms had persisted after age 16 years. Gittelman and her colleagues believed that it was the conduct or antisocial disorder, not the use of psychostimulants to control ADHD symptoms, that led to the development of substance abuse.

Although stimulants have a pronounced beneficial effect on ADHD symptoms in 70 percent to 80 percent of patients, children and adolescents treated with stimulants alone continue to have problems of poor school performance, low self-esteem, poor socialization, and poor behavior. A comprehensive treatment program, of which medication is just one aspect, is needed to address the serious accompanying problems of ADHD. Different types of treatment include family, individual, and group counseling, with a focus on improvement of the adolescent's social skills and impulse control. Special education needs will depend on whether poor academic performance has resulted from the ADHD symptoms or whether a learning disability is also present. Educational and social outcome is better when not only ADHD symptoms but also the various accompanying disabilities all receive therapeutic attention.

Conduct or Antisocial Disorder and Juvenile Delinquency

Antisocial disorder occurs in adolescents who have had a childhood history of conduct disorder. These two disorders are defined as sequential in DSM III-R, the onset of antisocial disorder being 18 years of age. Conduct disorders and antisocial disorders in turn are related to the legal entities of juvenile delinquency and adult criminality. These psychiatric and legal entities play an important role beginning in early adolescence because at this time the tolerated and less severe aggressive misbehaviors of childhood assume a more malignant nature. The progression from disruptive behavior to minor aggression to major aggression often occurs in the school setting.

Two factors are important in the psychiatric assessment of conduct disordered youth. First, these adolescents often have severe mental disorders in addition to their conduct disorder. Second, conduct disordered adolescents often have coexisting neuropsychological abnormalities. These two factors affect the clinical presentation of the conduct or antisocial disorder and may play an important role in treatment decisions.

Adolescents referred for evaluation of conduct or antisocial disorders may have severe emotional symptoms in addition to their more obvious conduct symptoms. These teenagers may manifest anxiety or depression. They may describe auditory or visual hallucinations and may demonstrate delusional or paranoid thinking. These psychotic symptoms may, however, have been obscured by concurrent alcohol or drug abuse.

Two important studies have helped to establish the association of conduct disorder and delinquency with psychotic symptoms. Bender (1959) described a group of psychotic children who went through an antisocial phase during adolescence. They showed behavioral symptoms such as violence, stealing, fire setting, and sex offenses. Upon psychiatric examination, these teenagers often demonstrated persistence of childhood symptoms of paranoid thinking, anxiety, and hallucinations. In the second study, published 23 years later, Lewis, Shanok, and Pincus (1982) described a group of violent and repetitively delinquent adolescents who lived in a correctional institution. Many youths in this group manifested paranoid symptoms, visual and auditory hallucinations, and rambling, illogical thinking. More psychotic symptoms were present in the more violent delinquents. In addition, in several cases the juvenile's psychotic thinking had influenced the performance of the violent behavior. In many of these youngsters, the psychotic thinking was periodic and, therefore, not always present during the psychiatric evaluation (Lewis and Shanok, 1978).

Another study of 71 delinquents determined that all had multiple DSM III diagnoses (McManus, Alessi, Grapentine, and Brickman, 1984). The principal diagnoses were borderline personality disorder (37 percent), major affective disorder (15 percent), substance/alcohol abuse (13 percent), conduct disorder (11 percent), other personality disorders (7 percent), schizotypal personality disorder (6 percent), and schizophrenia (4 percent). Substance abuse was present as a principal or secondary diagnosis in most of these patients, and most had experienced multiple psychosocial stressors, a breakup of the family having occurred in 72 percent of the population. These adolescents averaged four out-of-home placements prior to their incarceration, and 38 percent had a history of psychiatric hospitalization. It is, thus, clear that conduct disordered youth often have severe mental disorders as well.

The second feature of adolescents with conduct or antisocial disorder and juvenile delinquency that is important in psychiatric assessment is the high frequency of neuropsychological abnormalities in this group. Neuropsychological functions are brain functions that are involved in the integration of mental and physical processes. These functions include memory, spatial cognition, rhythmic sequencing, and fine motor skills. Neuropsychological functions are tested with test batteries such as the Halstead-Reitan Neuropsychological Battery (Reitan and Wolfson, 1985) or the Luria-Nebraska Neuropsychological Battery. (Golden, Hemmeke, and Purisch, 1980)

Visual-motor integration and coordination is an example of a neuropsychological function. It enables people to determine their physical location in space and the location of objects in relationship to other objects. An extreme visual-perceptual deficit might prevent a person from being able to distinguish the position of letters or words on a written page. The Bender Gestalt Test is commonly used to test visual-perceptual functioning. Abnormalities in visual-perceptual and in other types of neuropsychological functioning are commonly detected in brain injured adolescents and in adolescents with other forms of neurological impairment. These abnormalities are also present in adolescents with learning disabilities and ADHD.

A high prevalence of neuropsychological abnormalities has been detected in delinquent populations. Delinquents have also been found to have a high prevalence of major neurological abnormalities, complex partial seizure disorders, and abnormal EEGs (McManus et al., 1984). As a possible explanation for these findings of neurological dysfunction,

Lewis and colleagues (1982) have demonstrated that physical abuse and severe head and facial injuries are common in the histories of incarcerated delinquents.

How useful is this knowledge of the psychiatric and neuro-psychological status of violent delinquents to an understanding of the patients that psychiatrists see in psychiatric outpatient clinics? Although the multiple handicaps of violent delinquents may appear to have little applicability to psychiatric patients, this is not the case.

First, increasing numbers of youths with similar problems of aggressive conduct and other severe behavioral and emotional conditions are now being evaluated in mental health facilities. Sometimes the only factor that distinguishes these patients from delinquents is that the patients do not have juvenile justice records. There are many adolescent psychiatric patients with severe aggressive or repetitive misconduct, however, who do have both psychiatric and juvenile justice histories.

Second, increased awareness of the concurrent presence of psychiatric and neuropsychological disturbance with conduct or antisocial disorder will result in new treatment approaches for this challenging group of youths. Comprehensive treatment must include educational, psychiatric, neurological, and psychosocial components. Educational treatment should address neuropsychological deficits, such as memory impairment and poor visual-motor performance. Psychiatric treatment should emphasize effective therapeutic interventions and the use of medications that treat aggression and impulsivity. Carbamazepine, lithium, and propranolol are three medications currently being used in the treatment of aggression. In addition, the psychiatrist should pay close attention to accompanying mental disorders that may contribute to the youth's behavioral disorder. A neurological evaluation is necessary to document the presence of seizure disorders and other remediable neurological conditions. Further, psychosocial interventions must address environmental circumstances that contribute to the onset of conduct disorder. These environmental circumstances are well known and include poverty, broken families, parental mental illness, and poor parenting.

Most adolescents who qualify for school placements as emotionally handicapped also have conduct disorders. A student qualifies for a special education placement as emotionally handicapped when academic testing demonstrates a deterioration in school performance that can be attributed to the presence of a behavioral or emotional condition. The educational needs of students with aggressive conduct, however, are quite different from those of other students also designated emotionally handicapped, such as autistic students, for example. The behavior of aggressive adolescents must be controlled if they are to learn, whereas with autistic adolescents the educational focus is on fostering their communication skills and social interaction. Larger school systems can provide separate instruction for students with behavior disorders and those with emotional disorders. Smaller school systems, however, which have only a few children in a diagnostic category, may have to place children with different problems together.

Effects of Substance Abuse

Adolescents' experimentation with mind-altering, illicit drugs is so widespread in the United States that it has become normative behavior. Alcohol is the most frequently used mind-altering drug. The prevalence of teenage experimentation with alcohol in 1977 was about 70 percent (Blane and Hewitt, 1977). Furthermore, the incidence of lifetime illicit drug use has increased over the past 20 years, with the mean age of first use being 15 years by the late 1970s. Most concern is directed toward the 10 percent of adolescents who experiment with and then become dependent on alcohol or drugs. Dependency occurs when the person develops a physical or a psychological need for the drug and focuses great time and energy on drug-seeking activities.

Adolescents who use substances such as marijuana often differ in values and lifestyles from those who do not use substances (Kandel, 1982). For example, the school performance and academic interest of substance users frequently are lower. In addition, substance users are more often involved in delinquent acts and traffic violations and less often involved in religious activities.

A progression usually occurs in drug use, which begins with legal drugs and leads to illicit substances (Kandel, 1982). Adolescents usually try beer and wine first. Next they go to hard liquor and cigarettes. The next stage is marijuana use, which begins after the use of liquor or cigarettes. Problem drinking is next. The final stage is the use of illicit drugs other than marijuana. Adolescents who have progressed to illicit drugs are often abusing more than one substance, and the earlier any drug is used, the more likely it is that other drugs will be used.

Two currently held theories attempt to explain substance abuse in different ways. The self-medication theory (Khantzian, 1985) states that adolescents use drugs over long periods to treat feelings of psychological distress. Furthermore, these adolescents apparently are able to select the appropriate illicit drug to alleviate the type of distress they are experiencing. Paton, Kessler, and Kandel (1977) demonstrated that preexisting symptoms of depression are the primary predictors of subsequent marijuana use. Likewise, adolescents who use cocaine often report preexisting symptoms of chronic depression. Cocaine may transiently alleviate for these adolescents certain characteristics of

depression, such as fatigue or feelings of depletion. In addition to transiently relieving depressive symptoms, cocaine is also believed to lessen
inattention, distractibility, and impulsivity in adolescents who have
attention-deficit hyperactivity disorder. Individuals who abuse
morphine-like drugs may have preexisting psychoses or severe
aggressive behavior that they are attempting to treat.

The second theory that attempts to explain substance abuse does
not argue that abuse is related to preexisting mental disorders. Rather,
it views abuse as a habit disturbance, such as smoking, and as a
symptom of addiction, not as a symptom of an underlying mental disorder (Vaillant, 1980).

Many factors contribute to the risk of alcohol and drug abuse. Sex,
ethnic background, the presence of psychiatric disorders, and the abuse
of other drugs all play important roles, as do low self-esteem and personality traits such as aggressiveness and rebelliousness. Use of alcohol
and drugs by parents and peers also contributes to the likelihood that
an adolescent will abuse some substance. For example, almost all drug
addicts in Maryland come from families in which at least one parent
abused alcohol (*Baltimore Sun*, 1986). In addition, adoption and twin
studies give evidence for a hereditary component in alcoholism.

Chronic alcohol and drug use is maladaptive during adolescence.
Alcohol and drugs are used to avoid the stress and unpleasant feelings
that often accompany the events of adolescence. Thus, chronic users
do not develop the mature coping skills that result from mastering
stressful situations. Substance abuse may also lead to a lowering of self-
esteem, along with feelings of alienation and loneliness. In some adolescent drug users, an amotivational syndrome, characterized by apathy
and withdrawal from demanding social situations, will occur. Because
the stresses and tasks of adolescence are, as stated, particularly challenging for handicapped youth, these youngsters may be at high risk for
substance abuse.

Suicidal Behavior and Depression

The following case history of a 16-year-old adolescent girl, Lisa,
illustrates two more behavioral and emotional conditions commonly
seen in handicapped youth: suicidal behavior and a depressive disorder. In this instance, mental disorder led to a traumatic brain injury
and became a complicating factor in recovery.

Lisa was the fourth of four children and an eleventh grade student
in a vocational high school. Family history was notable in that Lisa's
father was alcoholic. The patient began to receive special education

services in the fourth grade when a reading disability was discovered. Lisa had been a loner in grade school and was often teased by classmates. Her mother recalls that Lisa did not feel attractive and that she lacked self-confidence. At age 13 years the patient and her mother saw a counselor several times because of the teasing at school. One year later Lisa saw a psychiatrist because of lack of involvement in her studies. No diagnosis was available from these two mental health interventions.

Lisa recalls that she had been depressed on and off for 2 or 3 years and first thought of committing suicide 1 year before she made the suicide pact that resulted in her injury. Lisa met John, a newcomer in her neighborhood, 6 months before they made the suicide pact. The pair saw each other on several occasions and agreed to kill themselves with a gun. Lisa shot herself in the back of the head and damaged her right cerebellum, a part of the brain regulating movement, balance, and speech.

Lisa remained comatose for 1 week. The patient's verbal and performance IQ returned to the low average range within 2 months. Persistent deficits were left-sided paralysis, impaired balance, and poor speech articulation.

Intermittent suicidal ideation persisted during recovery, and Lisa was admitted to a psychiatric hospital 3 months after her suicide attempt. During her stay she complained of feelings of depression but displayed little emotional response to important events in her life. She showed low self-esteem, was withdrawn from close personal attachments, and had impaired sleep and appetite. One month of inpatient treatment was followed by individual and family psychotherapy on an outpatient basis. Twelve months after her injury, Lisa was readmitted to the psychiatric hospital because of recurrent suicidal thinking. She complained of depressed mood, diminished interest in activities, decreased appetite, and poor sleep; she fulfilled DSM III-R diagnostic criteria for major depression. A combination of individual and family psychotherapy and antidepressant medication was successful in symptom reduction and in improvement of school and home adjustment over the following year.

Lisa's case illustrates several conditions: suicidal behavior, a depressive disorder, a learning disability, and traumatic brain injury. She probably had an incompletely treated depressive disorder at the time of her suicide pact. Although she had been teased and had low self-esteem since grade school, Lisa recalls the onset of her depression being about 13 years of age.

Suicidal Behavior

Suicide is currently the third most common cause of death in the 15- to 24-year-old population. The suicide rate in adolescence more than quadrupled from 1950 to 1980 and is now about 12 per 100,000 persons (Blum, 1987). The highest suicide rate is among white males. Nonfatal suicidal attempts are very common, especially among white females. For every 100 to 150 female adolescents who make a suicide attempt, one female adolescent succeeds. The rate for male adolescents is one completed suicide per 30 to 50 attempts.

Although there is little specific information about handicapped populations, current research is focusing on depression and suicidal behavior in nonhandicapped adolescents. Thus, there is increasing knowledge about risk factors, clinical course, and treatment of these conditions. Stressful childhood experiences are commonly noted in the history of suicidal adolescents (Pfeffer, 1985). These stresses include forms of family disruption such as death, divorce, separation, and birth of a sibling. Furthermore, certain emotional states and behavioral disorders are frequent in suicidal adolescents. These adolescents are likely to be depressed, as is illustrated by the case history of Lisa. Many are abusing drugs at the time they attempt suicide. Hostility, conduct problems, and aggressive behavior are also common in suicidal adolescents. In a study of 31 completed suicides of youngsters ages 12 to 14 years, 17 percent had conduct/aggressive problems, 57 percent had conduct/aggressive problems and were also depressed, and 13 percent had symptoms of depression (Shaffer, 1974).

Moreover, certain similarities characterize the environments of suicidal adolescents. Many have suicidal and depressed parents, and family violence is frequent. Those adolescents who have been physically or sexually abused are at high risk for the development of suicidal behavior, and often the abuse is the precipitant for the suicide attempt.

Imitation also plays a role in adolescent suicide attempts. This imitation may be a developmental factor related to the importance of peer influence during the adolescent years. These imitative suicides frequently share clinical characteristics with the isolated suicides discussed earlier, however. Studies have documented an increased number of teenage suicides after broadcast of television shows about suicide (Gould and Shaffer, 1986; Phillips and Carstensen, 1986). Teenage suicides may also cluster in a certain school or area over a short period of time. The case history of Lisa illustrates another form of peer influence, the suicide pact. In such instances two socially isolated people develop an emotional closeness and share a delusion of pessimism and hopelessness. This delusion leads to the creation of the suicide pact.

Depression

Symptoms of depression are common during adolescence. In one sample of 385 junior and senior high school students, 13.5 percent were mildly depressed, 7.3 percent were moderately depressed, and 1.3 percent were severely depressed (Kaplan, Hong, and Weinhold, 1984). In another sample that applied DSM III criteria to teenagers in a community, depression was the third most prevalent psychiatric disorder; it was found in 2.7 percent of the boys and in 13.3 percent of the girls (Kashani et al., 1987). The criteria for adolescent depressive disorders are nearly the same as those used for children and adults. Age-specific features are listed for certain depressive disorders in the DSM III-R. For example, sulkiness, school difficulties, and feelings of not being understood are adolescent features of a major depressive episode. More of these age-specific features will undoubtedly be included in future diagnostic manuals as adolescent depressive symptoms are clarified in clinical studies.

Diagnosis of adolescent depression is not easy, and this has led to both underdiagnosis and overdiagnosis of the condition. Some adolescents are not introspective and are unable to talk about their inner feelings. Others overestimate the degree of their depression. When adolescents are interviewed with their parents, often there is disagreement about the degree of depression that is present. Furthermore, there are times when depression is diagnosed with little clinical evidence, but it is assumed that the adolescent must be depressed because of his or her poor environmental circumstances.

It is important to inquire about all symptoms of depression, as well as about the level of academic and social functioning. Self-rating scales may be helpful in considering a range of symptoms. A number of self-rating scales, such as the Beck Depression Inventory and the Depression Self-Rating Scale, are in current use. Teenagers often readily accept these scales as an objective way to help define the problems they are having. Both scales can be used reliably in adolescents who have a verbal IQ of 55 or above (Beck, Carlson, Russell, and Brownfield, 1987).

There are two main ways to treat adolescent depression: psychotherapy and drug therapy. At times these forms of treatment are used together to achieve maximum treatment benefit. Treatment studies of adolescents are limited thus far, and information about various treatments therefore often is obtained from adult studies. Generally, mild forms of depression tend to be treated with psychotherapy, whereas more severe forms are treated with a combination of psychotherapy and drug therapy.

Most adolescents receive psychotherapy for their depressive disorders. Cognitive therapy and interpersonal therapy are two types of psychotherapy that have been beneficial in both depressed adults and adolescents. Cognitive therapy is an active form of therapy in which patients are confronted about their negative views of themselves and their environment. They are then presented with a more orderly, consistent, and self-corrective approach to dealing with their problems (Hodgman, 1985). Interpersonal therapy concentrates on the resolution of problems in the patient's relationships. Family therapy, which may include individual psychotherapy of other family members, is also an important treatment for adolescent depression.

Although antidepressant medication is now being used widely in the treatment of adolescent depression, studies that actually demonstrate its therapeutic benefits are lacking (Rifkin, Wortman, Reardon, and Siris, 1986). Also, teenagers with bipolar disorder do not appear to respond as well as adults to treatment with lithium. Future clinical studies will clarify these diagnostic and treatment issues.

It is clear, then, that care must be exercised in the use of antidepressant medications with adolescents. When these drugs are indicated, they should be prescribed in limited quantities to depressed teenagers, as suicidal youngsters may use them to make suicide attempts. (See Chapter 4 for further discussion of the antidepressant medications.)

SUMMARY

The incidence of death and illness among adolescents in this country was 11 percent higher in 1986 than it was in 1976 (*American Medical News*, 1986, p. 3). Many of the topics discussed in this chapter—violence, substance abuse, suicide, teen pregnancy, and traumatic injury—are major contributing factors. Prevention and treatment programs focusing on these urgent adolescent problems must acknowledge the special needs of handicapped adolescents and modify services as necessary to serve this population.

REFERENCES

Alan Guttmacher Institute. (1985). *Fact sheet.* Planned Parenthood Federation of America, Inc., U.S. Department of Health and Human Services. December 1, pp. 1–5.

American Medical News, December 19, 1986. AMA launches teen health project, p. 3.

American Medical News, December 19, 1986. An urgent need in adolescent health care, p. 4.

Baltimore Sun, December 13, 1986. Treatment for the addict, p. 10.

Beck, D.C., Carlson, G.A., Russell, A.T., and Brownfield, F.E. (1987). Use of depression rating instruments in developmentally and educationally delayed adolescents. *Journal of the American Academy of Child and Adolescent Psychiatry, 26,* 97–100.

Bender, L. (1959). The concept of pseudopsychopathic schizophrenia in adolescents. *American Journal of Orthopsychiatry, 29,* 491–509.

Blane, H.T., and Hewitt, L.E. (1977). *Alcohol and youth. An analysis of the literature, 1960–1975.* Springfield, Virginia: National Institute on Alcohol Abuse and Alcoholism, National Technical Information Service. NIAAA Contract 281-75-0026.

Blum, R. (1987). Contemporary threats to adolescent health in the United States. *Journal of the American Medical Association, 257,* 3391–3395.

Chess, S., Fernandez, P., and Korn, S. (1980). The handicapped child and his family: Consonance and dissonance with special reference to deaf children. *Journal of the American Academy of Child Psychiatry, 19,* 56–67.

Chilman, C. (1983). *Adolescent sexuality in a changing American society.* New York: John Wiley and Sons.

Gilchrist, E., and Wilkinson, M. (1979). Some factors determining prognosis in young people with severe head injuries. *Archives of Neurology, 36,* 355–359.

Gilchrist, L.D., and Schinke, S.P. (1983). Counseling with adolescents about their sexuality. In C.S. Chilman, *Adolescent sexuality in a changing American society* (pp. 230–250). New York: John Wiley and Sons.

Gittelman, R., Mannuzza, S., Shenker, R., and Bonagura, N. (1985). Hyperactive boys almost grown up: 1. Psychiatric status. *Archives of General Psychiatry, 42,* 937–947.

Gittelman-Klein, R. (1987). Prognosis of attention deficit disorder and its management in adolescence. *Pediatrics in Review, 8,* 216–222.

Golden, C.J., Hemmeke, T., and Purisch, A.D. (1980). *The Luria-Nebraska neuropsychological battery manual.* Los Angeles: Western Psychological Services.

Gould, M.S., and Shaffer, D. (1986). The impact of suicide in television movies. *New England Journal of Medicine, 315,* 690–694.

Grob, C. (1986). Substance abuse: What turns casual use into chronic dependence? *Contemporary Pediatrics, 3,* 26–41.

Hodgman, C.H. (1985). Recent findings in adolescent depression and suicide. *Developmental and Behavioral Pediatrics, 6,* 162–170.

Kandel, D. (1982). Epidemiological and psychosocial perspectives on adolescent drug use. *Journal of the American Academy of Child Psychiatry, 21,* 328–347.

Kaplan, S.L., Hong, G.K., and Weinhold, C. (1984). Epidemiology of depressive symptomatology in adolescents. *Journal of the American Academy of Child Psychiatry, 23,* 91–98.

Kashani, J.H., Beck, N.C., Hoeper, E.W., Fallahi, C., Corcoran, C.M., McAllister, J.A., Rosenberg, T.K., and Reid, J.C. (1987). Psychiatric disorders in a community sample of adolescents. *American Journal of Psychiatry, 144,* 584–589.

Khantzian, E.J. (1985). The self-medication hypothesis of addictive disorders: Focus on heroin and cocaine dependence. *American Journal of Psychiatry, 142,* 1259–1264.

Lewis, D.O., and Shanok, S. (1978). Delinquency and the schizophrenic spectrum of disorders. *Journal of the American Academy of Child Psychiatry, 17,* 263–276.

Lewis, D.O., Shanok, S., and Pincus, J. (1982). A comparison of the neuropsychiatric status of female and male incarcerated delinquents: Some evidence of sex and race bias. *Journal of the American Academy of Child Psychiatry, 21,* 190–196.

Lussier, A. (1960). Analysis of a boy with a congenital deformity. *The Psychoanalytic Study of the Child, 15,* 430–453.

McManus, M., Alessi, N., Grapentine, W.L., and Brickman, A. (1984). Psychiatric disturbance in serious delinquents. *Journal of the American Academy of Child Psychiatry, 23,* 602–615.

Myers, B.A. (1987). Psychiatric problems in adolescents with developmental disabilities. *Journal of the American Academy of Child and Adolescent Psychiatry, 26,* 74–79.

Offer, D. (1987). In defense of adolescents. *Journal of the American Medical Association, 257,* 3407–3408.

Oldham, D. (1978). Adolescent turmoil–a myth revisited. *Adolescent Psychiatry, 6,* 267–279.

Paton, S., Kessler, R., and Kandel, D. (1977). Depressive mood and adolescent illicit drug use: A longitudinal analysis. *Journal of Genetic Psychology, 131,* 267–289.

Pfeffer, C.R. (1985). Self-destructive behavior in children and adolescents. *Psychiatric Clinics of North America, 8,* 215–226.

Phillips, D.P., and Carstensen, L.L. (1986). Clustering of teenage suicides after television news stories about suicide. *New England Journal of Medicine, 315,* 685–689.

Reitan, R.M., and Wolfson, D. (1985). *The Halstead-Reitan neuropsychological battery: Theory and clinical interpretation.* Tucson: Neuropsychology Press.

Rifkin, A., Wortman, R., Reardon, G., and Siris, S. (1986). Psychotropic medication in adolescents: A review. *Journal of Clinical Psychiatry, 47,* 400–408.

Satterfield, J.H., Hoppe, C.M., and Schell, A.M. (1982). A prospective study of delinquency in 110 adolescent boys with attention-deficit disorder and 88 normal adolescent boys. *American Journal of Psychiatry, 139,* 795–798.

Shaffer, D. (1974). Suicide in childhood and early adolescence. *Journal of Child Psychology and Psychiatry, 15,* 275–291.

Vaillant, G.E. (1980). Natural history of male psychological health: VIII. Antecedents of alcoholism and orality. *American Journal of Psychiatry, 137,* 181–186.

Weiss, G. (1983). Long-term outcome: Findings, concepts, and practical implications. In M. Rutter (Ed.), *Developmental Neuropsychiatry* (pp. 422–436). New York: The Guilford Press.

Zabin, L.S. (1986). The school based approach to teen pregnancy prevention. *Planned Parenthood Review, Spring,* 8–10.

Zabin, L.S., Hirsch, M.B., Smith, E.A., Strett, R., and Hardy, J.B. (1986). Evaluation of a pregnancy prevention program for urban teenagers. *Family Planning Perspectives, 18,* 119–126.

CHAPTER 4

MEDICAL TREATMENT OF PSYCHIATRIC DISORDERS IN HANDICAPPED CHILDREN

Lea O'Quinn

T he medical treatment of psychiatric disorders in handicapped youngsters begins with a complete psychiatric evaluation. As was described in Chapter 2, this process results in a DSM III-R diagnosis (American Psychiatric Association, 1987), which is preliminary to treatment planning. The results of the evaluation, including the diagnosis and a formulation of the patient's problem, provide a rationale for treatment and lead the psychiatrist to certain treatment alternatives. These treatments include various types of psychotherapy, behavioral therapy, the use of medication, and combinations of these treatment methods.

PSYCHOTHERAPY

Depending on the psychiatric diagnosis, the child's level of intellectual functioning, and the effect of family stresses, a determination is made about the usefulness of individual, family, or group psychotherapy or combinations of these.

Individual Therapy

Individual therapy can take the form of play or talking, or it can be a combination of these two. Some individual psychotherapy is time limited and goal specific; some is more open ended. Therapy can be supportive or directive, geared toward problem solving or achieving insight. All individual therapy, however, provides youngsters with an outlet for expressing their thoughts and feelings and provides them with an opportunity to explore alternative thoughts and behaviors. The goal is to help children develop an increasing sense of their own ability to be autonomous, caring, and competent people. Psychiatrists, child psychologists, mental health workers, and social workers are the professionals trained to conduct individual therapy with children.

Play is often used by these therapists to evaluate children's attention span, their affective states, and their fine and gross motor functioning. Therapists may then use the play to help children improve their self-concepts through success experiences or explore alternatives to certain patterns of behavior. Affective states such as anger, sadness, and fearfulness may be demonstrated by children in play, and these feelings can be named by the therapist to help children recognize what they are experiencing. These feelings can be understood and supported in the context of the play. Alternative scenarios can be constructed by therapists that allow children to gain a sense of control and mastery over these feelings.

The dollhouse is a useful tool for allowing children to demonstrate their understanding of day-to-day occurrences within their family. The therapist can gain a sense of how interactive the family is, how organized, and how supportive from the child's point of view. Furthermore, as children play with the dollhouse, they can depict their own feelings: their sense of isolation, sadness, anger, fearfulness, or anxiety. For example, children who are angry or have lived in a chaotic, hostile environment often demonstrate aggression in their play. Children who are sad and isolated and who feel unloved will demonstrate this in their play with the dolls. In the dollhouse of such a child, people don't eat or talk together. One doll may always be alone even when other family members are together. Children who are anxious will demonstrate their attempts to find safety or to escape frightening situations. Superheroes, police, or doctors are often called on to rescue them. Not infrequently, children will demonstrate a sense of hopelessness, and no one can help them. The therapist can then use the play to introduce options and to offer the child choices about how things might turn out. Puppets can also be used in play to help the child demonstrate feelings, thoughts, and actions.

Drawings are often used in play therapy, as are games and building toys. In the course of play, the therapist can help the child develop social skills, such as turn taking, good sportsmanship, and consideration for others. Children learn these skills through the example of the therapist, and they then practice them. The goal is for children to use these interactions with peers and family and thus to improve their own self-concepts. Play can also be used to decrease the sense of isolation some children have and to teach them, if necessary, how to deal with name calling or teasing. Physically handicapped children can learn how to respond more adaptively to being looked at, and they can learn how to handle misconceptions and questions about their conditions.

Sometimes during individual therapy sessions, children play with toys such as building blocks or puzzles while they talk. This situation may be less anxiety provoking for them than just sitting and talking with the therapist. The use of a tape recorder can also be helpful. Children tell their stories into the recorder, and the therapist and child can then use the tape as they construct other possible meanings, scenarios, and outcomes.

The ideal individual therapy situation occurs when the child is able to talk to the therapist like an adult. In these cases, toys or props are not necessary. Many children, however, are unable to talk directly with the therapist about their problems and thus need games or other play materials to help them express their thoughts and feelings.

Family Therapy

Family therapy may be the recommended treatment for some handicapped children's disorders and is often helpful to other family members as well. Parents, the affected child, and siblings all have feelings about their situation that affect the interactions among family members. Patterns of interaction develop that may not be conducive to growth, but until the feelings and behaviors can be explored in family sessions, little change can occur. Often family members are unaware of the existence of these patterns, or if they are, they do not see them as problems. It is only when individual members can be heard by the whole family that change may be possible.

In families that function well, parents are in charge, have a strong parental coalition, and share responsibilities in agreed-upon ways. They are sensitive to their children's needs, and they avail themselves of support from extended family and community and friends. Children in such families feel the strength and fairness and sensitivity of their parents and are able to grow as individuals, participating in school, making friends, and pursuing individual interests. This kind of family functioning, however, may be more difficult to achieve when one member of the family is handicapped, but it is possible. The following case history illustrates a family with a handicapped child that functions very well.

Audrey was a child who was born with congenital rubella, which resulted in congenital heart disease and a severe hearing impairment. She also had visual impairment and functioned in the borderline range of intelligence. During the early years of her life, she required multiple hospitalizations for correction of the heart defect. Simultaneously, attention was focused on helping her cope with the hearing and visual impairments. She was fitted with glasses and hearing aids and she, her parents, and her younger brother all learned a combination of sign language and lip reading. Audrey was also enrolled in classes for the hearing impaired.

Early in her life Audrey's parents were sensitive to the need for social interaction, and they looked for opportunities for special classes providing mainstreaming. This was difficult. In spite of the requirements of Public Law 94-142 (Palfrey, Morris, and Butler, 1978), which mandates schools to provide for the needs of handicapped children, the schools in this family's state could not provide the specific educational programs that the parents were convinced that Audrey needed. Their school system offered an alternative program, but the parents did not find it acceptable. Rather than fight with the schools, the parents found in another state the program they thought was the most conducive to their daughter's growth, and they moved there. Audrey's mother became a teacher of the deaf, and her father found suitable employment in the new state. Audrey's brother started school there, and Audrey mastered sign language and lip reading and communicated with a combination of sign and talking.

All seemed to go well until Audrey, at the onset of puberty, developed behavioral problems at home and at school. She became hostile and aggressive. During a psychiatric interview, with the parents at times serving as interpreters, Audrey spoke with emotion of the social isolation she felt. Nonhandicapped peers could not understand her when she spoke; they called her "dummy." Hearing impaired peers could understand her, but when they were together in public places and communicated by signing, people stared at them, and she felt self-conscious and embarrassed. She was sad, frustrated, and angry.

The parents, who together had fought the system to provide for opportunities for Audrey to be as normal as possible, were frustrated and angry about the way the world had responded, and they questioned what they could do. But they worked together on the problem and were sensitive to the needs of both of their children for progress toward independence. They came to therapy as a family to present their problems, to grieve the circumstances, to consider alternatives, and to seek support. They encouraged their son to con- tinue activities with friends and school, and they opened their home to their children's friends. They found ways for their daughter to participate more in age-appropriate activities that were safe and could help her to become more independent. These included more mainstream classes, Girl Scouts, and interactions with peers in the neighborhood. As Audrey's sense of competence improved in somewhat sheltered activities, her anxiety, sadness, and anger decreased, and the stress level in the family also decreased. The support the parents gave each other, their sense of a common goal for their children, and their willingness to accept help from the outside permitted them to work together and to meet the challenges presented to them. There will be more challenges in the future; however, this family's ability to deal with Audrey's adolescent behavior problem attests to their ability to cope well with adversity and bodes well for the future.

The case example of Audrey illustrates successful use of family psychotherapy and successful family adaptation to the problems presented by having a handicapped child. In other families with a handicapped child, however, less positive patterns of interactions may occur. Individual and family therapy can also help in these cases, as the following case history illustrates.

Melissa was an $11\frac{1}{2}$ year old youngster who was well until 7 years of age, when she was found to be in congestive heart failure after suffering from myocarditis, a viral inflammatory process affecting the heart muscle. Her course over time was difficult, with multiple hospitalizations and progressive decompensation in cardiac functioning. Although Melissa had been an independent child, after the onset of this illness her tolerance for exercise became limited. This caused her parents to worry about her health and stamina, and they became more protective of her. The parents had previously had some marital difficulties and had avoided dealing with these by not talking about them.

When Melissa's mother did not see any improvement in her condition, she began to limit Melissa's activities more and more, and the father disagreed with these limitations. They did not discuss this, however. Rather, the parents, in essence, just agreed to disagree. The mother became more and more aligned with the daughter, insisting that the girl not go anywhere unless she was with her. She did not permit Melissa to ride her bicycle except in front of the house and enrolled her in a home-bound school program. Melissa's mother arranged for the grandmother to quit her job and care for Melissa in the day time.

Melissa began sleeping with her mother. Her siblings, an older brother and a younger brother, complained about the attention that Melissa received, and at times they were required to stay with her rather than going out to play. The father began spending less and less time at home, ostensibly to earn more money so that medical expenses for Melissa could be covered. When he was home, he was irritable and angry. He began drinking heavily. Melissa stayed close to her mother "to protect" her from her father. In this context, she was admitted to the hospital in congestive heart failure, fearful of being separated from her mother, and "hysterical" about having medical procedures performed.

During an interview with the psychiatrist, Melissa was sullen and initially refused to talk. After 2 weeks of individual and group therapy, she was able to talk about her worries about family finances, her brothers' complaints, her mother's welfare, and her father's behavior. She was able to express her anger about the restrictions on her life. She could appreciate that they had come about out of caring on the part of her mother. She wanted to be free to ride her bicycle around the neighborhood just as her brothers did, however. She wanted to ride the school bus like other children, and she wanted to be able to go places with her friends and without her mother. She was tired of waking up from a nap to find her mother peering at her in tears.

One day she asked to have a family meeting to tell her parents all of this. She was anxious and repeatedly asked for support. In the family meeting, she demonstrated remarkable caring, self-assurance, a sense of humor, and strength. She clearly told her parents about all the issues she had planned to discuss. Her wisdom was remarkable. At one point her mother said, "I've just wanted to be sure you were safe." To this Melissa replied, "Life means taking risks. You're not giving me a chance to live." When she told her father about his behavior, she said, "I don't like the things you do; you scare me." Initially he was defensive, saying, "Well, adults have a right to do some of those things." Later he was able to say he understood why Melissa found him to be "scary" at times, but he was also able to tell her that he would like to have her sleep back in her own bed so that he could sleep in his. The session ended with the parents planning to consider together how they might respond to Melissa's request for more independence. They also agreed to bring the siblings for the next session as a prelude to ongoing family meetings at home, another of Melissa's requests. Melissa also stated she was willing to undergo cardiac catheterization, a procedure she had previously refused.

This case history shows the usefulness of psychotherapy for resolving family conflicts. In this family, Melissa's strength, which was present before her illness, was rekindled through individual, group, and family therapy. This permitted the parents to consider the maladaptive patterns of interaction that had developed over the years and worsened in the context of their anxiety about Melissa.

Melissa's case history makes an important point. Children with handicaps can also have enormous strengths. It is important to recognize these so that they can be used for growth.

USE OF MEDICATIONS

Medication is an important medical therapy for children and adolescents with mental disorders. Psychiatric medications are used to treat certain symptoms, such as hyperactivity, hallucinations, inattention, depressive mood, and poor appetite. No current pediatric medication relieves all symptoms of a disorder or eliminates any disorder. For this reason, medication is usually not effective as the only treatment for a mental disorder. When it is combined with other forms of treatment, such as psychotherapy, social work, and special education, maximum therapeutic benefit may result for the child or adolescent.

Several different classes of medications may be helpful in the treatment of psychiatric disorders in handicapped youngsters. The use of these medications should be undertaken with full knowledge by parents and the child about how they might be helpful, about interactions with other drugs the child may be taking, and about side effects; parents and child should be partners with the psychiatrist or physician. This partnership requires that the doctor present parents with all relevant information. The parents must feel free to ask questions about the medicines suggested and to inquire about other medications they have heard about. Such full disclosure and discussion is necessary to determine what is helpful for the child. Sometimes parents are very trusting and will do whatever the physician suggests, and sometimes physicians are paternalistic, believing that they know what is best and that their judgments should not be questioned. Neither of these situations is conducive to the family's growth. The physician can present options and recommend a course of action. It is up to the family, however, to decide which they will select. That decision will be based on their level of trust, their financial resources, the availability of care, and the information available to them. There is no one "right" way to proceed. What is most helpful for families is to maintain a sense of autonomy, an ability to negotiate, and a feeling of confidence that they have chosen the best options for themselves. This keeps the family involved in a way that permits them to be of most help to their handicapped child and allows them to be free enough to pursue other aspects of life as well. In short, a physician-family partnership promotes everyone's growth.

In a discussion of the use of medications for psychiatric disorders in handicapped youngsters, either the classes of medications or the types of disorders for which medications may be helpful might be discussed. In this chapter, the disorders for which medications may be helpful are described. Difficulties encountered in making certain diagnoses, particularly in the handicapped, and about the side effects of commonly used medications are also addressed.

MENTAL DISORDERS AND THEIR MANAGEMENT

Attention-deficit Hyperactivity Disorder (ADHD)

This disorder, characterized in children by symptoms of inattention, impulsivity, and hyperactivity, has been the most frequently diagnosed neurobehavioral disorder in childhood. (See also Chapters 2 and 6.) The prevalence rates of ADHD average between 5 and 10 percent of all children, with boys being affected more often than girls by ratios of 3 or 4 to 1. The cause of ADHD is unknown, but hereditary influences are thought to play an important role. In some children with ADHD, the neurological examination reveals the presence of "soft signs" or neuromaturational delay. These include difficulties with the establishment of consistent laterality and some problems with fine and gross motor coordination. These are not signs of major neurological impairment or signs of a structural nervous system abnormality, and they are not present in all children with ADHD. On physical examination, some children with ADHD demonstrate minor signs of physical malformation, such as low-set ears, which are usually of no clinical significance. By and large, most children with ADHD have normal physical and neurological findings on examination.

Once the evaluation of children with ADHD is complete, including psychological and educational testing, their management often includes the use of medication. Furthermore, an appropriate educational placement is needed that provides structure and freedom from distractions. Some children may need a curriculum geared to helping them with specific learning problems. In addition, the family often needs supportive counseling to help them deal with their feelings about their child's behavioral difficulties. Moreover, they may well benefit from working with a therapist versed in behavior management techniques. Such a therapist can help parents set up a system so that the child learns that appropriate behavior will be rewarded and unacceptable behavior will have consequences that are known and fair. The child with speech and language impairment will also need appropriate services. When a team of clinicians works together in the management of children with attention-deficit hyperactivity disorder, the team members attend to these children's multiple needs and systematically monitor their progress. The following case history is illustrative.

Brian was a 9-year-old youngster who was referred for evaluation and treatment of poor academic performance and school misbehavior. At home, he was pleasant but had difficulty following through on directions and expectations. On physical examination, Brian was noted to have poor hygiene, to be small for his age, and to be fidgety and talkative. Neurological examination revealed some difficulties with fine motor coordination. During the interview, his speech was clear, without articulation difficulty, and he appeared to function in the borderline range of intelligence. Brian's language was rambling, and his answers to questions were not to the point. He expressed fearfulness and awe about phenomena such as monsters and the devil. He denied experiencing hallucinations and delusions and denied specific phobias.

Psychological evaluation confirmed the presence of borderline intelligence, with academic functioning two to three grade levels behind in all subjects. Brian was highly distractible and had difficulty concentrating. A language evaluation further defined his problems with staying on the subject and responding appropriately to questions. During more extensive psychiatric evaluation, Brian demonstrated both oppositional disorder and overanxious disorder. He talked of having been physically abused and said that he feared being abandoned. His stepfather drank and fought with his mother, and on occasion they sent him and his siblings to spend the night away from the house. During these times, he was particularly worried about his mother's welfare and about himself as well.

Brian was started in a remedial education program with few classroom distractions, and he was enrolled in group and individual therapy and language therapy. His parents became involved in family therapy. When Brian failed to show significant progress over the first 4 to 6 weeks of treatment, an antianxiety medication was added to the other therapies. The safety of the home was also evaluated by the Department of Social Services, and a behavioral program for home use was instituted. Some improvement occurred over the next month in that Brian demonstrated less fearfulness and anxiety in the individual sessions. However, school distractability continued, and Brian made little progress in his language therapy. The diagnostic possibility of attention-deficit hyperactivity disorder was then considered, and the antianxiety medication was discontinued.

The following week, Brian was started on a stimulant, methylphenidate (Ritalin), with resultant marked improvement. This improvement occurred both in classroom performance and in his language therapy. As Brian experienced success, he became more self-assured and was able to comply better with the behavioral system. He appeared less anxious.

Brian's case history is characterized by a complicated psychiatric picture, which could only be understood after an extended evaluation. This child had several problems associated with his poor school performance: neurological, cognitive, language, and emotional. Each of these problems had to be addressed before significant improvement could occur. Brian's academic and language performance were useful in monitoring the benefits of medications.

Stimulants

The stimulants are a class of drugs that have been used for years in treating children with a variety of behavioral difficulties. At the present time the main clinical use of the stimulants is with children diagnosed as having attention-deficit hyperactivity disorder. Stimulant medication decreases symptoms of inattention, impulsivity, and hyperactivity in children with this disorder. It is unclear whether stimulants have a positive long-term effect on learning. The effect of stimulants is not specific for ADHD, however, and these medications have similar behavioral effects on children without mental disorder. Three drugs will be considered here: dextroamphetamine, methylphenidate, and pemoline sodium.

Dextroamphetamine (Dexedrine) was originally described by Bradley (1937) as a drug that could be helpful in children with a combination of learning and behavioral problems. It was found to be a medication that could help children focus their attention and therefore be less distractible and less impulsive. Thus, behavior could be improved, and the child could attend better to what parents and teachers were trying to teach. A second drug, *methylphenidate (Ritalin)* was found to have similar properties and has also been used in helping children focus attention. Both dextroamphetamine and methylphenidate begin to act about 30 minutes after administration, with the peak action being about 2 hours after administration. Methylphenidate is metabolized and no longer exerts a therapeutic effect after about 3 to 6 hours. Typically these medications are administered in the morning before school. Some children require a second dose around noon to maintain attention during the entire school day. In some children who take dextroamphetamine or methylphenidate, a worsening of symptoms of hyperactivity, inattention, and impulsivity is seen as the effects of the medication wear off. This is sometimes referred to as a "paradoxical rebound." A third drug, *pemoline sodium (Cylert)* has similar therapeutic properties and can be given once a day rather than in multiple doses because its duration of action is longer than that of the other two drugs.

In recent years, a long-acting form (sustained release) of methylphenidate (Ritalin SR) has been developed and can also be given once a day. This long-acting medication has two advantages: (1) Children do not have to take medication again at midday, and (2) this drug has a smoother onset and decline of action. Some children, however, do not respond as well to the long-acting preparation as they do to the short-acting dextroamphetamine or methylphenidate.

DOSAGE OF STIMULANTS. Determination of dosage of the stimulants typically is made on the basis of the child's response; that is, the decision is an empiric one. Sprague and Sleator (1977) have suggested that these drugs' effects on behavior and attention span depend on dosage. They found that with lower doses of methylphenidate (0.3 mg/kg) there was more improvement in performance on attentional tasks, whereas at higher doses (1 mg/kg) there was more improvement in activity level.

As a general rule, the dose of dextroamphetamine is half that of methylphenidate. Typically, the initial dosage for children of dextroamphetamine is 2.5 mg given in a single dose or 2.5 mg given twice a day. The comparable dosage of methylphenidate is 5.0 mg given in a single dose or 5.0 mg given twice a day. Occasionally, these medications are given three times a day. Dosages and times of administration are adjusted to achieve an optimal clinical response, with careful attention given to the appearance of side effects. Some children do very well on the smaller doses, e.g., 5.0 mg of methylphenidate given in a single dose or 5.0 mg given twice a day. On occasion, doses higher than 20 mg per day of methylphenidate may be needed.

With the long-acting stimulants, such as pemoline sodium or Ritalin SR, the dosage also needs to be adjusted. The initial dosage of pemoline sodium is usually 37.5 mg. This can be increased by a half tablet, or 18.75 mg, at weekly intervals, until the desired effect of improved attention span is achieved or until it is determined that the medication is not helpful. The usual dosage of pemoline sodium is 56.25 to 75 mg daily. For the sustained release methylphenidate, the single morning dose is usually the total of the individual doses utilized with the regular methylphenidate. For example, if a child were taking 10 mg twice per day, then the dosage of the SR form would be 20 mg in the morning.

Once a beneficial dose is arrived at, the child is maintained at that dose until it is determined that the medication is no longer needed or that a change in dosage is indicated. As discussed in Chapter 3, these medications continue to be effective during adolescence. While children are on medication, they can learn to increase their attention spans and decrease impulsivity through behavioral means. It may well be that they can then use these behavioral methods to sustain the desired behaviors, and the medication will no longer be necessary. The decision to stop the medication is based on how the child does during drug holidays. These can occur on weekends and during vacations from school.

SIDE EFFECTS OF THE STIMULANTS. The stimulants have known and predictable side effects, depending to some extent on dosage. That is, the lower the dosage, the less the likelihood that side effects will occur. Among the more common side effects are (1) decrease in appetite, (2) interference with initiating sleep, and (3) increase in heart rate and blood pressure (usually of no clinical significance). Children on pemoline sodium should be followed periodically with blood tests of liver function, as there have been reports of liver dysfunction in patients taking this medicine.

Growth suppression related to total dosage is an important side effect of stimulant medication. One study has demonstrated significant but small decreases in both weight and height percentiles occurring during methylphenidate administration (Mattes and Gittelman, 1983). The decrease in weight percentiles occurred from the first year of treatment, whereas the decrease in height percentiles was apparent after 2 to 4 years of treatment. To address this problem, dosage reduction and drug holidays are recommended with stimulant use, because when the dosage is reduced or the drug is temporarily stopped, there is often a period of increased or catch-up growth.

Some children develop tics (involuntary, repetitive, purposeless, rapid motor movements or vocalizations) while taking stimulant medication. These tics may be transient, lasting only a short time, or they may be chronic, lasting for a year or more. Sometimes, while taking stimulants, children develop a combination of motor and vocal tics, called Tourette's syndrome. It is advisable to discontinue the stimulant when a tic appears. It is also generally advisable to avoid stimulant use when children have close relatives with tics or Tourette's syndrome.

Major Depression

The evaluation of children for symptoms of depression has in recent years come under careful scrutiny. The symptoms of the depressive disorders are discussed in Chapter 2. In handicapped youngsters, symptoms of major depression may be difficult to ascertain. These children may not be able to describe their feelings of sadness and hopelessness, and, if they have a significant motor handicap, they may not be able to demonstrate their feelings in play. Thus, the family and the psychiatrist may have to decide about the presence of depression on the basis of facial expression, tearfulness, or a change in behavior. For example, significant symptoms may include the onset of sleep difficulties that persist and that are accompanied by increased or decreased activity levels. Irritability, crying spells, a decreased ability to concentrate, a decline in school performance, and a lack of interest in surroundings are other meaningful symptoms.

Antidepressants have been used successfully to treat major depression in nonhandicapped children and should be considered in the treatment of handicapped children as well. Whether or not antidepressants are used, psychotherapy should be included in the treatment regimen. The following cases histories of two handicapped youngsters with major depression are illustrative.

Paul was a 14-year-old youth who was born with multiple congenital anomalies, among them a cardiac malformation (ventricular septal defect). Early in his life, surgical repair was attempted and was successful, but resulted in a complication: complete heart block. This then required the placement of a pacemaker. At the time of this evaluation, Paul had been admitted for replacement of his pacemaker, which had begun to malfunction. Other pertinent past history is that he had had surgery on three occasions for repair of hypospadias, a urinary tract anomaly, and the surgery had not been successful. One and a half years prior to this hospitalization, he had been treated for scoliosis, curvature of the spine, with surgery and the placement of a Harrington rod. One year prior to the present admission, because of threats of self-harm, he had been hospitalized for 1 month for the treatment of major depression and subsequently was being seen by a child psychiatrist once a month as an outpatient. He had progressed as an average student in school until recent months.

A psychiatric evaluation was requested because when he was hospitalized for the replacement of his pacemaker, he refused to have the procedure performed. The mother revealed that her son had demonstrated "a change in personality" after the scoliosis surgery $1\frac{1}{2}$ years earlier. Before the surgery he had been talkative and fun loving, but since that time he had been irritable and argumentative. Although the mother believed the psychiatric hospitalization and outpatient follow-up subsequent to the scoliosis surgery were helpful, she had not seen her son return to his "old self" after discharge from the hospital. Rather, he had continued to be irritable, argumentative, and unhappy.

During the interview with the psychiatrist, Paul appeared as a sullen boy who was small for his age, although pubescent, and who spoke with an articulation disorder. At times it was difficult to understand what he said. He actually said little spontaneously, and he avoided eye contact. Paul had coarse facial features and joint malformations of the fingers of both hands. His affect was irritable, although he denied feeling sad, angry, or anxious. Paul's behavior was impulsive and unpredictable, and at one point during the interview he angrily threw his slipper across the room. He denied any problems with appetite but did state that he had difficulty getting to sleep and that sometimes he would awaken in the middle of the night and have difficulty going back to sleep. He denied experiencing hallucinations and delusions, and denied being phobic except about medical procedures. He claimed he was frightened about needles in particular, and that was why he was refusing to have the pacemaker replaced. Over the next 24 hours, during discussions with family members, he decided to undergo the pacemaker replacement surgery.

Paul and the family were told that he had symptoms of a major depression, and medication was recommended. After the pacemaker replacement, he was started on imipramine (Tofranil), an antidepressant. The plan was formulated for Paul to be seen by a behavioral psychologist for desensitization to medical procedures, but this was not initiated during the short hospital stay. Furthermore, evaluations were undertaken, including metabolic studies and chromosome studies, to try to find the cause of his multiple congenital anomalies. He was subsequently followed by his outpatient psychiatrist, and his mother reported improvement in his mood. She was beginning to see signs of Paul's "old self" after he was on imipramine for 3 weeks.

Paul will need to continue in outpatient psychotherapy, in which he can address numerous issues of adolescence, including identity, self-concept, and independence. Furthermore, desensitization to medical procedures is also needed because Paul will have to undergo surgery in the future for repair of the hypospadias and replacement of the pacemaker. His willingness during this admission to undergo evaluation to find the cause of his multiple congenital anomalies should help him begin to better accept and cope with these handicaps.

Paul's case illustrates the effective use of antidepressant medication with a handicapped 14-year-old boy. Carol's case, described next, required no antidepressants but rather other medical and psychiatric interventions.

Carol was 21 years old at the time of referral. She had been found at 9 years of age to have a brain tumor (a craniopharyngioma). She was operated on successfully and did well educationally and socially until she was 16 years of age, at which time a recurrence of the tumor necessitated a second operation.

After her second surgery, Carol demonstrated learning and memory problems and experienced difficulty in completing high school. It was hard for her to follow directions, and her social judgment was poor. After high school she was unable to obtain employment, and at home she became progressively more irritable and aggressive. Carol's appetite and food intake increased, and she gained 25 to 30 pounds in the 6 months before her admission.

At the time of hospitalization, Carol was found to be functioning in the borderline range of intelligence, with marked difficulty in short-term memory. A CT scan showed no recurrence of tumor.

During the interview with the psychiatrist, Carol appeared as a sad but cooperative young lady who fulfilled DSM III-R criteria for dysthymia, a chronic disturbance of depressed mood. She spoke poignantly of her memory of herself as someone who functioned well in school and with her peers. She cried frequently as she talked of her isolation at home and her desire to be a woman who could have a job and who could become a mother. She stated that becoming a mother had always been very important to her, and she had come to feel that it would never happen. The one person she had dated several years before had recently married, and furthermore she had had problems with her menstrual period. She had suffered hormone imbalance related to the brain surgery and was of the opinion that she would feel better if she could have regular menstrual periods.

Upon discussion with Carol, her physician, her parents, and the psychologist, the following plan was developed. She was put on replacement hormones to achieve some regularity in her menstrual periods. She was enrolled in outpatient therapy at the local mental health center so that she could talk about her worries and frustrations and receive support and intervention. She was put on the waiting list for participation in the adult day program at the mental health center so that she could begin to be more involved in the outside world. Her mood and her behavior improved on the basis of these interventions. Antidepressant medication was not believed to be indicated, as Carol's mood disturbance had responded so quickly to these other therapeutic measures.

Antidepressants

The *antidepressant* that has been used most widely in children for the treatment of depression is imipramine (Tofranil). The names of other antidepressants which have been used in treating childhood depression are desipramine (Norpramin), nortriptyline (Aventyl, Pamelor), and amitriptyline (Elavil). When consideration is being given to using antidepressants for the treatment of depression in children, parents must be fully informed about the risks and benefits. When antidepressants are used in children, the indication for their use and a detailed management plan must be carefully documented.

DOSAGE OF ANTIDEPRESSANTS. Psychiatrists can use the child's weight in choosing the initial dose of antidepressant, (giving a certain number of milligrams per kilogram), or they can begin with a standard, commonly used dose. In either case, the dose is further adjusted by periodic blood level determinations of the drug. Each of the antidepressants mentioned earlier appears to have a therapeutic range of blood level that needs to be achieved for the medication to be effective but not toxic (Task Force on the Use of Laboratory Tests in Psychiatry, 1985). For example, imipramine therapy in children is usually started with a dosage of 25 mg at bedtime, increasing to 50 mg over the first few days. A blood level is then obtained to determine whether additional drug is needed to achieve the therapeutic range. Once the therapeutic range is reached, blood levels should be checked periodically to ensure that the proper level is being maintained. In adults and, it seems, in children as well, it may take as long as 3 weeks at therapeutic level to begin to get a therapeutic response. As some children appear to metabolize the drug rapidly, it is best to give it in two to three divided doses during the day. The dose at bedtime is sometimes helpful in relieving sleep disturbance before the other therapeutic effects occur. Usually antidepressants in children are continued for 6 to 8 months, after which time the dose is gradually tapered over a 2-week period, and the medication is then discontinued.

SIDE EFFECTS OF ANTIDEPRESSANTS. Children may experience dry mouth, constipation, and urinary retention as side effects of antidepressant medication. More serious, however, are the side effects of cardiac toxicity. For this reason it is important not only to monitor blood levels, but also to have periodic electrocardiograms. Some children and adults may also experience orthostatic hypotension when on these medications, causing them to feel faint if they stand up from a sitting position too rapidly. For this reason, blood pressure monitoring in both sitting and standing positions should occur at periodic intervals, and adjustments should be made in the dosage or timing of medication to minimize this side effect. Another helpful maneuver is to teach the patient to get up slowly from a sitting position rather than changing abruptly.

The child's physical condition must be considered when the possibility of depression is evaluated. Illness or handicap may play a significant role in causing a depression, as was seen in the case histories of Paul and Carol. Also, knowledge of the child's physical condition before the use of medication is helpful in determining the presence of side effects.

Bipolar Disorder or Manic Depressive Illness

Bipolar disorder, commonly referred to as manic depressive illness, is a mental disorder that is characterized by one or more manic episodes, usually with a history of depressive episodes. The disorder is frequently seen as an inherited condition. During manic periods, the patient demonstrates an elevated, expansive, or irritable mood. During the depressed periods, the patient is sad, has low energy level, and feels down in the dumps and blue. Between the episodes of heightened and depressed moods, periods of normal mood may occur for months at a time. Psychotic symptoms (the presence of hallucinations and/or delusions) may occur in conjunction with the disorder of mood.

Only recently have symptoms of mania been recognized in children. Careful evaluation over time may be required as the symptoms of mania are at times hard to distinguish from the symptoms of attention-deficit hyperactivity disorder, particularly in handicapped youngsters. The diagnosis can be made, however, by keeping careful behavioral records and observing changes in mood from expansive to more subdued over certain time periods. Mood is usually elevated, and the activity level is usually high. The child is more talkative and distractable than usual, and there is often a heightened interest in sexual matters. Sleep is disturbed, and it is hard for these children to get settled for bed.

Medication for Bipolar Disorder

Lithium is the drug used most frequently in the treatment of bipolar disorder or manic depressive illness. In adults it has been found to be very helpful in achieving stability of mood over time. Because the symptoms of mania have been recognized to exist in children only recently, the use of lithium in children has not been widespread.

Carbamazepine (Tegretol), a drug used primarily as an anticonvulsant, has been used as an alternative to lithium for the treatment of bipolar disorder or manic depressive illness in some adult patients. In children it may be a useful alternative for the treatment of mania when the occurrence of side effects, such as frequent urination and bedwetting, precludes the continued use of lithium. When psychotic symptoms accompany the mood disturbance, treatment with neuroleptics may be indicated. The neuroleptics, or major tranquilizers, are discussed in greater detail later in this chapter.

DOSAGE. The dosage of lithium is determined by the patient's blood level evaluation. The patient begins with 300 mg daily and usually increases to 300 mg twice a day given with meals to prevent gastric irritation. Several days later, a blood level is obtained, and the dosage is adjusted so that the blood level ranges between 0.8 and 1.2 mEq/liter. It may take up to 1 week at therapeutic blood levels to observe a therapeutic effect.

The dosage of carbamazepine is determined by blood level as well. Typically, children begin with a dosage of 100 mg twice a day and increase by 100 mg per day to a dose of 400 mg per day. A blood level is then obtained, and the dosage is adjusted to achieve a blood level that is within the therapeutic range for anticonvulsant treatment.

SIDE EFFECTS. Before therapy with lithium is undertaken, an EKG and renal and thyroid function tests should be done. While the patient is on lithium, these tests should be repeated periodically. Side effects, which can occur when the blood level climbs above the therapeutic range, may include nausea and vomiting, drowsiness, and problems with coordination. If the dosage is not adjusted, toxic symptoms affecting neurological function occur, resulting in progressive difficulties in coordination, seizures, stupor, and coma. Thus, it is very important to monitor blood levels to ensure that they stay within the therapeutic range. During the summer, children on lithium should be monitored carefully for toxicity, because as sodium is lost in sweat, more lithium is absorbed for the dose administered, and this may result in higher blood levels.

Side effects of carbamazepine include blood, kidney, and liver toxicities. Therefore, children on carbamazepine should be evaluated before starting the drug and periodically thereafter with complete blood counts and tests of renal and liver function.

Pervasive Developmental Disorders (PDD)

Pervasive developmental disorders are a group of disorders in which multiple aspects of a child's development are impaired. Such children are especially handicapped in the use of language and in social interactions. The cause of these disorders remains unknown but appears to be related to organic factors.

Autistic Disorder

Autistic disorder is the most severe form of pervasive developmental disorder. Autistic children often are noted to be different from the time of birth. They tend to be temperamentally difficult, with little desire for cuddling, and are irregular in their times for eating and sleeping. They tend to avoid eye contact from infancy and seem to be in their "own world," with little interest in interpersonal contact and stimulation. They may achieve motor milestones at expected times. Language acquisition is often markedly delayed, however, and when it is acquired, it is often characterized by such abnormalities as repetitive speech (echolalia) and idiosyncratic use of words. Autistic children tend to have a short attention span for learning and at the same time to perseverate in activities in which they are absorbed. These activities appear to be self-stimulatory and include rocking, looking at lights in various ways, and engaging in repetitive motor acts, such as spinning wheels or twirling tops. At times the repetitive behaviors are self-injurious, such as head-banging or scratching.

The level of intellectual functioning of autistic children affects their ability to learn and their ultimate overall level of functioning. Some autistic individuals function in the average range of intelligence, and a few are college graduates. Even these, however, show a scatter in cognitive abilities with deficits in comprehension, judgment, and abstract reasoning. They may have excellent visual-spatial and memory skills, however. Most (about 75 percent) function in the moderate range of mental retardation and below. All autistic children are in need of special educational attention from the preschool years onward, along with close collaboration between teachers and parents to address academic performance, social behavior, self-help skills, and language development.

A few autistic children become more interested in social interaction as they become adolescents. This is especially true of those who function closer to the average range of intelligence. It is difficult in these autistic adolescents to modulate their interest in other people, and they are often seen as socially intrusive. They may get too close to other people physically, and they often ask intrusive questions or make comments that are socially offensive. For example, they may ask strangers about their parentage, their academic performance, their dating or other aspects of their social life, or their religious beliefs. Thus, comprehension of social situations and judgment remain markedly impaired. It is these deficits that are handicapping in the late adolescent and early adult years and that hamper progress in achieving independent employment and living arrangements.

The following case demonstrates the difficulties encountered at times in managing a child with autistic disorder. What is used as a tool to help the child in one developmental stage may become a problem later on, a problem that continues to hamper growth toward independence. (For a detailed discussion of the educational management of children with pervasive developmental disorders, see Chapter 7.)

John, an autistic 17-year-old who functioned in the average range of intelligence, had spent a considerable amount of time watching TV during his early years. He was not talking then, and he was especially interested in TV commercials, which he at times imitated. His favorite commerical was one for women's hose, and the staff at his day care center used this interest to teach him language by exposing him to hose and by telling him and showing him about hose. He did begin talking, and his interest in hose also continued. As he grew, he developed a habit of sleeping with hose and an interest in wearing them himself. The latter behavior was discouraged. In spite of admonitions to the contrary, John became socially intrusive with girls and women as he approached adolescence. He would get close to them and then slip his hand down to touch their hose. Needless to say, this behavior was inappropriate and served to distance him from young women, some of whom were so surprised and offended that they considered reporting him to the police.

In therapy sessions, John expressed concern about making friends, having a girlfriend, and getting married and having children. Guidelines were established with him about appropriate social behavior, about how to make friends, and about behavior with girlfriends. He was enrolled in a sex education course and given advice about not getting married until he was 22 years old and had a job. In addition, a behavioral program was initiated to decrease his interest in touching hose. In spite of these measures, John continued to be socially and sexually inappropriate. After consultation with representatives of a sexual disorders clinic, he was enrolled in group therapy and was also started on Depo-Provera, a female hormone that has had some success in decreasing sex drive in men. Subsequently he showed improvement in being more appropriate in his behavior with women. However, side effects of the medication, which included significant weight gain and some hypertension, resulted in its discontinuation.

It is possible that John would have become sexually intrusive at puberty whether or not he had developed this early interest in hose. It appears, however, that the early preoccupation with hose, which was used successfully to help him establish communication, later contributed to his socially inappropriate behavior and became an additional handicap.

Medication for Pervasive Developmental Disorders

Some children with pervasive developmental disorders and autistic disorder may be helped by medication. Neuroleptics or major tranquilizers are a group of medications that may be beneficial in the treatment of these disorders. These medications are most effective in reducing symptoms of hyperactivity, agitation, and aggression. They also reduce self-injury, stereotypic behavior, and angry affect in this group of children (Campbell, 1985). In one group of 40 autistic children, haloperidol (Haldol) was effective in reducing stereotypic behavior, withdrawal, hyperactivity, and poor interpersonal relationships (Anderson et al., 1984). These medications are always used in combination with other forms of treatment, such as behavioral therapy and special educational methods to obtain the best possible outcome.

Neuroleptics may be differentiated on the basis of potency, sedative properties, and other side effects. A smaller dose of a high potency drug is needed to achieve the same therapeutic result as a larger dose of a low potency drug. For example, a haloperidol (high potency neuroleptic) dose of 2.5 mg is equivalent to a 100 mg dose of thioridazine (low potency neuroleptic). High potency neuroleptics tend to be less sedating and have less anticholinergic side effects (constipation, urinary retention, dry mouth), but more extrapyramidal effects. Extrapyramidal effects include certain motor phenomena, such as stiffness of movement, involuntary muscle contractions, and akathisia, a feeling of restlessness and an urge to pace. Extrapyramidal side effects can be relieved through the use of anticholinergic medications such as diphenhydramine (Benadryl) and benztropine (Cogentin).

Haloperidol (Haldol), trifluoperazine (Stelazine), and fluphenazine (Prolixin) are examples of high potency neuroleptics with few anticholinergic side effects. Fluphenazine decanoate (depot Prolixin) is an injectable, long-acting neuroleptic that can be used for noncompliant patients. These three drugs are unlikely to cause sedation and orthostatic hypotension. Patients on these drugs are more likely to develop the extrapyramidal motor effects discussed previously, however. Thioridazine (Mellaril) and chlorpromazine (Thorazine) are examples of low potency neuroleptics that more frequently cause anticholinergic side effects and orthostatic hypotension. Extrapyramidal side effects are less common with this group of neuroleptics.

Neuroleptics should be used and monitored with great care, because their long-term use can result in tardive dyskinesia, an irreversible movement disorder involving chiefly the cheeks, lips, and tongue, but on occasion other body parts as well. Tardive dyskinesia becomes apparent when neuroleptic medication is discontinued. There is no known treatment for tardive dyskinesia, so it is important to limit as much as possible the dose and duration of neuroleptic treatment. In some patients, a temporary movement disorder, withdrawal dyskinesia, is seen at the time that the neuroleptic is discontinued. This withdrawal dyskinesia can last for as long as 4 months and then remit (Gualtieri, Shroeder, Hicks, and Quade, 1986). Any dyskinesia persisting for longer than this period of time after withdrawal of neuroleptics is considered to represent tardive dyskinesia. An Abnormal

Involuntary Movements Scale (AIMS) should be performed before, during, and after neuroleptic treatment to monitor the emergence of involuntary movements. Parents need to be fully informed about the.risk of tardive dyskinesia and informed consent should be obtained.

In children, the high-potency neuroleptic medications tend to be used in dosages of from 1 to 20 mg per day, whereas the low potency medications are usually prescribed in doses from 10 to 300 mg per day.

Mental Retardation

Mental retardation is the term applied when individuals are found to function in the subnormal range of intelligence on standard measures of adaptive and cognitive functioning. This mental handicap results in a slower rate of learning, and the affected person is impaired in most aspects of cognitive development. Thus, special education arrangements are needed, and families must adjust to the idea that their child is retarded and to the child's special needs.

Being retarded imposes additional risks for psychiatric disorder (Szymanski and Tanguay, 1980). The term "dual diagnosis" has been used to designate those individuals who not only are retarded but who also have additional behavioral or emotional handicap. These individuals with dual diagnosis require particularly careful evaluation and treatment so that they can achieve and maintain their best levels of functioning.

A disproportionate number of mildly retarded people come from families that are chaotic and occasionally abusive. The realization that this was the case provided an impetus for the development of the multiple early intervention programs of the 1960s and 1970s. Coming from difficult home settings and experiencing frustration at school, these mildly retarded individuals are at risk for developing a number of psychiatric disorders, including depressive disorders and adjustment disorders. The following case history is illustrative.

> Larry, a 10-year-old boy who functioned in the mild range of mental retardation, was referred for evaluation and treatment of aggressive and self-injurious behavior. Because of his behavior, he had been removed from his most recent foster home and was living in an emergency shelter. His mother was retarded, his father was alcoholic, and his parents were separated. Two older brothers had served time in prison for assault and larceny, a sister was in foster care, and another brother had drowned accidently 2 years before.
>
> The members of this multiproblem family were known to the schools and social agencies of their town as "troublemakers." Representatives of the agencies saw Larry as a born troublemaker, and they were unable to find a foster home or a suitable classroom

placement for him. A young social worker, new to the community, was assigned to Larry's case and brought him for evaluation.

During the interview, Larry avoided eye contact and appeared sad. His talk was difficult to understand because of an articulation disorder. There was no evidence of language disorder in the brief answers he gave to questions, however. He stated that he had frequent crying spells and had difficulty sleeping. In addition, Larry stated that he had thought about killing himself. He spoke of feeling responsible and guilty about his brother's death. He claimed to hear his dead brother talking to him and telling him to come to be with him. He denied, however, experiencing delusions or phobias.

Larry was considered to have major depression and to be experiencing auditory hallucinations related to that depression. Owing to concerns about his safety, he was hospitalized and was treated with antidepressant medication. During the hospitalization, he responded well and was successful in the structured classroom setting. He received articulation therapy and the clarity of his speech improved. He responded well to a behavior modification program, which succeeded in decreasing the frequency of his aggressive and threatening behavior. He stopped hearing voices, his mood improved, and the suicidal ideation was no longer present. Larry was discharged to a group home, and on follow-up over the next 4 months he was doing well.

Larry's case demonstrates the importance and benefits of determining the reasons for behavioral difficulties in individuals who are mentally retarded. In Larry's case, his behavioral problems were related to his depression, which in part was due to his chaotic family situation.

Psychotic Symptoms

Psychotic symptoms in children are characterized by the presence of delusions and certain kinds of hallucinations that indicate a loss of touch with reality. They can occur as part of delirium, major depression, a manic episode, schizophrenia, and also in situations of severe stress.

Childhood hallucinations are often innocent, as when a child hears his or her name called aloud or when a deprived child hallucinates the vision of a wished-for toy. The psychiatrist must determine if the child's hallucinations indicate a psychotic process. For example, in children, auditory and visual hallucinations can occur in the context of a major depression. In this circumstance, the hallucinations have a depressive theme, such as voices telling the child he is bad and that he should step out in front of a car or jump out of a window. Such hallucinations are dangerous because they are continuous and compelling.

Delusions are fixed, false beliefs, and may be persecutory (individuals believe there is a plot against them) or megalomaniacal (individuals believe they have special powers, talk with God, are the King or Queen of England). Delusions also may be of control (individuals believe their thoughts are not their own and are controlled by others) or depressive (individuals believe their body is rotting or they are responsible for all the starvation in the world). Delusions are uncommon in childhood.

Treatment

Effective treatment of psychotic symptoms consists of identification and treatment of the underlying mental disorder. Psychotic children may have to be hospitalized to protect them from their own threatening hallucinations and delusions. If a child has a depressive or manic disorder with hallucinations, treatment would be a combination of psychotherapy and appropriate medication. If a child has symptoms of schizophrenia, then treatment with neuroleptic medication and psychotherapy is indicated. A hallucinating youngster with a brief reactive psychosis may respond to psychotherapy alone or to a combination of medication and psychotherapy.

Delirium is a mental disorder characterized by impaired attention and disorganized thinking, along with other symptoms, such as reduced level of consciousness, disorientation, and memory impairment. It can be caused by electrolyte imbalance and central nervous system infection, and it can also be seen as a side effect of medication. Delirious children are best treated by correction of the underlying problem, although a low dose of a major tranquilizer is sometimes helpful. In addition, having familiar people around and keeping a light on at night are helpful in the treatment of delirium.

SUMMARY

In this chapter, some of the most common psychiatric disorders have been described, with particular emphasis on their manifestations in children with handicapping conditions. The medical treatments of these disorders, which may include psychotherapy and medication, are discussed and illustrated with case histories.

REFERENCES

American Psychiatric Association. (1987). *Diagnostic and statistical manual of mental disorders* (3rd ed.—revised). Washington, DC: Author.
Anderson, L.T., Campbell, M., Grega, D.M., Perry, R., Small, A.M., and Green,

W.H. (1984). Haloperidol in infantile autism: Effects on learning and behavioral symptoms. *American Journal of Psychiatry, 141,* 1195-1202.

Bradley, C. (1937). The behavior of children receiving Benzedrine. *American Journal of Psychiatry, 94,* 577-585.

Campbell, M. (1985). Schizophrenic disorders and pervasive developmental disorders/infantile autism. In J.M. Wiener (Ed.), *Diagnosis and psychopharmacology of childhood and adolescent disorders* (pp. 114-150). New York: John Wiley and Sons.

Gualtieri, C.T., Schroeder, S.R., Hicks, L. and Quade, D. (1986). Tardive dyskinesia in young mentally retarded individuals. *Archives of General Psychiatry, 43,* 335-340.

Mattes, J.A., and Gittelman, R. (1983). Growth of hyperactive children on maintenance regimen of methylphenidate. *Archives of General Psychiatry, 40,* 317-321.

Palfrey, J.S., Morris, R.C., and Butler, J.A. (1978). New directions in the evaluation and education of handicapped children. *New England Journal of Medicine, 298,* 819-824.

Sprague, R.L. and Sleator, E.K. (1977). Methylphenidate in hyperkinetic children: Differences in dose effects on learning and social behavior. *Science, 198,* 1274-1276.

Szymanski, L.S., and Tanguay, P.E. (1980). *Emotional disorders of mentally retarded persons.* Baltimore: University Park Press.

Task Force on the Use of Laboratory Tests in Psychiatry. (1985). Tricyclic antidepressants—blood level measurements and clinical outcome: An APA task force report. *American Journal of Psychiatry, 142,* 155-162.

CHAPTER 5

BEHAVIORAL APPROACHES TO THE ASSESSMENT AND TREATMENT OF HANDICAPPED CHILDREN AND ADOLESCENTS

John M. Parrish and Thomas M. Reimers

The prevalence of behavior disorders among children with chronic mental or physical handicaps is well documented (Matson and Mulick, 1983). Disobedience, disruption, aggression, property destruction, and self-injury are but a few of the many problems that may hinder a handicapped child's functioning. Such behavior may place the child, as well as his or her peers and caregivers, at considerable risk and may interfere with medical treatment or educational programming. In fact, behavior disorders may even shift the focus from trying to help the child to a more normal lifestyle to simply maintaining him or her in a highly restrictive, nontherapeutic environment. Recurrence of behavior problems is a frequent cause of school or job failure and is often a primary factor in considering alternative educational, work, or residential placements, some of which may be less than ideal for the handicapped youngster.

Assessment and intervention strategies based on the principles of applied behavior analysis have proved to be cost-effective methods of addressing behavior disorders among handicapped children and adolescents. Applied behavior analysis is the area of scientific activity concerned with the development of practical procedures for producing changes in human behavior (Baer, Wolf, and Risley, 1968). Strategies based on applied behavior analysis have been shown to be effective in helping handicapped persons acquire and maintain the skills they need for optimal functioning.

Applied behavior analysis, sometimes called behavior modification or behavior therapy, has two defining characteristics. First, it examines and attempts to change what people say or do. Beliefs, attitudes, and feelings are important elements of the human condition. How these translate into action is the principal concern here. Second, applied behavior analysis contends that a person's behavior is a function of his or her environment, rather than of his or her intrapsychic drives, impulses, needs, motives, conflicts, or traits. Rather than viewing behavior disorders as manifestations of underlying emotional disturbances, mental diseases, or personality conflicts, applied behavior analysts believe that most behavior problems are learned and can be modified through learning procedures. Three types of learning are considered to be particularly critical in developing and changing behavior: classical or respondent conditioning (Pavlov, 1927), operant conditioning (Skinner, 1953), and observational learning (Bandura, 1969). Extensive descriptions of these learning theories are provided by Bandura (1977), Catania (1984), Hilgard and Bower (1966), Honig and Staddon (1977), and Kanfer and Phillips (1970).

This chapter provides an overview of the basic principles and methods of applied behavior analysis, with an emphasis on operant conditioning procedures. This is followed by an explanation of the steps typically taken by applied behavior analysts as they design behavior assessment and treatment programs for handicapped children. Next, the concerns of parents and teachers who work with behavior analysts are examined briefly. Finally, issues that arise when integrating behavior methods with medical or educational strategies are also explored. Throughout the chapter, case illustrations and recommended additional readings are offered to facilitate use of the information presented here.

PRINCIPLES AND METHODS

Positive Reinforcement

Applied behavior analysts often devise strategies to increase the frequency (or rate) of appropriate behavior among handicapped persons. Such methods are referred to as reinforcement procedures. *Reinforcement* refers to the presentation of an object or event following a behavior that will increase the rate or the probability that the particular behavior will occur in the future (Alberto and Troutman, 1982; Miller, 1980). Reinforcers can be social events, activities, manipulable objects, or edible items. Table 5-1 gives examples of reinforcers that are often presented to handicapped children or adolescents. The list of potential reinforcers is nearly endless and will vary from person to person.

TABLE 5-1.
Examples of Reinforcers for Handicapped Children and
Adolescents

Social Reinforcers
  Praise
  Gesture of approval
  Drawing closer to child
  Offering assistance when requested
  Asking about items or topics of interest
  Asking for demonstration of a skill already mastered
  Casual conversation

Activity Reinforcers
  Extra play period
  Caring for pets
  Going outside
  Passing out reinforcers
  Watching television
  Solving a puzzle
  Answering a telephone
  Going to a restaurant
  Listening to music

Manipulable Reinforcers
  Pencils, pens, and crayons
  Small toys (e.g., dolls)
  Grooming aids (e.g., combs and makeup)
  Musical instruments
  Games
  Money
  Tickets to special events
  Certificates of accomplishment
  Balls
  Magazines, books

Edible Reinforcers
  Raisins
  Carrots, celery
  Popcorn
  Dry cereals
  Fruit
  Crackers
  Chips
  Juice or soft drinks
  Ice cream
  Cookies

Planned Ignoring

Although reinforcement procedures are intended only to increase appropriate behavior, they may also inadvertently increase inappropriate behavior. For example, a parent who attends to a crying child may be increasing the likelihood the child will use crying in the future. A teacher who scolds a disruptive child may be reinforcing the disturbing behavior. Indeed, many children behave inappropriately to get some form of attention. If children continue to receive reinforcement for their misbehavior, it is likely that their poor conduct will continue or actually increase. In such situations, a procedure called *planned ignoring* has been shown to be effective in decreasing the rate of the problem behavior (Kazdin, 1984). Often referred to as extinction, planned ignoring is a technique that withholds reinforcement after the target inappropriate behavior (the behavior to be changed) occurs. In other words, a reinforcer that had previously followed the occurrence of a misbehavior is withdrawn.

Consistent ignoring of a child's nagging, whining, or crying, for example, will usually result in a decrease in these annoying behaviors. The desired effects of planned ignoring often are not immediate, however. Planned ignoring frequently produces an increase in the rate of the target behavior before a reduction occurs (Watson, 1967). This is known as an extinction burst. Another phenomenon that is likely to occur is referred to as spontaneous recovery (Skinner, 1953). This involves the reappearance of the undesirable behavior sometime after it has been extinguished. In this case, the handicapped child tests whether the planned ignoring is still in effect. The caregiver's continued ignoring of the behavior typically results in a rapid decrease in the behavior, however.

For example, consider a toilet-trained toddler who routinely cries when he awakens during the night. The parents have frequently responded to the crying by going to the child's room, removing him from bed, providing a cup of warm milk, and rocking him until he falls asleep again. If the parents were to employ planned ignoring, they would cease these reinforcing activities and instead do the following: (1) Quietly open the door to the child's room and determine whether the child is safe; (2) if the child is safe, close the door, and return to bed. The parents would not enter the child's room. At first, the child would probably cry for an extended period of time. If the parents consistently followed the planned ignoring procedure, however, the crying would gradually decrease, and the child would learn to return to sleep quietly. Every so often, the child may cry on awakening just to see if his parents will come to his rescue.

Differential Reinforcement

More often than not, a child will have several inappropriate behaviors that have been targeted for change, as well as several appropriate behaviors that require ongoing reinforcement. Consequently, positive reinforcement and planned ignoring are often combined in a procedure referred to as *differential reinforcement*. The objective of this procedure is to reinforce appropriate behavior while at the same time ignoring inappropriate behavior. Teachers employ a differential reinforcement strategy when they ignore a handicapped student who is talking out of turn, and then pay attention to this same student when he or she raises a hand to answer a question. Parents who ignore their children's tantrums but praise them when they play cooperatively are also employing differential reinforcement.

Differential reinforcement is preferred over planned ignoring because it indicates to a handicapped youngster which behaviors are appropriate and which are not. A key consideration when using differential reinforcement is to ensure that the inappropriate behavior is not acknowledged by someone else. For instance, a teacher may systematically ignore a particular child's inappropriate behavior, but that child may be receiving reinforcement from classmates or other adults during other times of the day in different settings. Consistent application of differential reinforcement by numerous caregivers across diverse settings often is required for behavior change to occur.

Shaping

In some situations the desired behavior may not be present in the child's repertoire at all, thereby providing no opportunity to reinforce the appropriate behavior differentially. The desired behavior may have to be developed or formed through a procedure called *shaping*. Shaping involves reinforcing selected behaviors in the individual's repertoire that resemble the target behavior. In this process, successive approximations to the target behavior are reinforced (Sulzer-Azaroff and Mayer, 1977).

To illustrate, consider teaching a handicapped youth to shoot a basketball. The instructor would first teach prerequisite skills, such as how to stop dribbling, how to grip the basketball when shooting, how to position the body for a shot, how to pinpoint the basket, and how to deliver a shot in proper form. Once such basic mechanics have been taught, the youth would practice shooting from a very short distance until several baskets were scored. The youth would then be directed to move back a few steps and so on until he or she is able to shoot accurately from desired distances.

In this example, the target behavior is accurate shooting from many different locations on the court. The successive approximations consist of first shooting accurately from short and then from longer distances. Accurate shooting at each court location is reinforced differentially by praising baskets made and ignoring baskets missed. This sort of shaping is often employed to help handicapped students learn new skills or behaviors.

Instructional and Imitation Training

Two other procedures are also commonly used to teach new behaviors. One is referred to as *instructional training* and involves describing a new behavior to the child. The other is termed *imitation training* and involves demonstrating the new behavior.

In instructional training, a teacher or parent describes what the child is to do, tells the child to perform the task, and then provides reinforcement to the child for following the instructions (Miller, 1980). Instructional training is used typically to teach new behaviors to children who have a sufficient receptive vocabulary. If a child's receptive vocabulary is deficient, imitation training, a strategy that relies less on a child's verbal skills, may be employed.

In imitation training, a teacher or parent demonstrates what the child is to do or learn, asks the child to imitate the behavior, and then provides reinforcement for the successful imitation of that behavior (Miller, 1980). For example, a teacher might use imitation training to teach a new word to a child. First, the teacher pronounces the word. Once the child has learned to imitate the word, the teacher can pair the expressed word with the actual object. For example, a teacher might say the word ''hair'' while pointing to her hair. This can be repeated until the child begins to touch his or her own hair (or the teacher's) while saying the word ''hair.''

Negative Reinforcement

Negative reinforcement, like positive reinforcement, is a procedure that is used to *increase* the frequency of a behavior. Negative reinforcement occurs when, as a result of a person's particular behavior, an aversive event is removed, which results in an increased rate of that behavior in the future. Put differently, a behavior has been negatively reinforced if its rate of occurrence increases because an aversive stimulus was withdrawn (Sulzer-Azaroff and Mayer, 1977). Examples of negative reinforcement are found commonly in our daily lives. We move inside to avoid the cold, stop at a red light to avoid a traffic accident, and take off a shoe to remove a pebble.

Negative reinforcement is frequently in operation at home and school, and it may increase undesired behaviors as well as desirable ones. Parents frequently reduce or remove punishment from their children to stop their nagging or complaining. For example, a parent may reduce a child's "grounding" from 3 days to 1 day to stop the child's whining about it. As a result, however, the child's whining is likely to increase. Another example of negative reinforcement occurs when parents finally remove the spinach the child has complained about eating. That is, they remove the aversive stimulus (spinach) as the consequence of a particular response (complaining). This results in an increase in that response in the future (complaining about spinach).

Punishment

Unlike positive and negative reinforcement, punishment refers to doing something following a behavior in order to decrease the rate or probability that the behavior will occur in the future. Punishment takes two forms: punishment by presentation and punishment by withdrawal. The former refers to the presentation of a punisher following the occurrence of a behavior. For example, a teacher may give a child a low grade on a paper to decrease poor performance in the future, or send a child to the principal's office as a result of an inappropriate behavior. A parent might punish by spanking a child for breaking a window, assigning extra household chores for being verbally abusive, or by scolding a child who is running toward the street.

Punishment by withdrawal refers to the removal of reinforcement. For example, a parent might withdraw the privilege of watching a favorite television show for lying, take away a child's play privileges for failing to complete homework, or remove a favorite toy for having a tantrum. A teacher might withhold recess from an aggressive student or restrict access to a special activity for an entire class because of its failure to follow a classroom rule.

Applied behavior analysts, however, have tended to avoid the use of punishment for several reasons: (1) There are a number of reinforcement-based approaches that can be used instead of punishment, (2) punishment can result in several negative side effects, (3) punishment procedures can be misused (Kazdin, 1984). Nevertheless, the application of punishment procedures is sometimes necessary. The ethical and effective use of punishment strategies is considered later in this chapter.

BEHAVIOR ASSESSMENT

The applied behavior analyst uses a combination of assessment approaches to identify behavior disorders in handicapped children. Among these approaches are structured interviews with parents or others, administration of rating scales or questionnaires to the same informants, and direct observations of the child in interactions with these key persons. During structured interviews with parents, teachers, or residential center staff members, the behavior clinician first obtains a global account of the caregiver's concerns. Checklists such as the Eyberg Child Behavior Inventory (Eyberg, 1980), the Behavior Problem Checklist (Quay and Peterson, 1979), and the Child Behavior Checklist (Achenbach and Edelbrock, 1979) are often integrated into the interview to help caregivers express and prioritize their concerns.

Defining Target Behaviors

Detailed assessments of the highest priority behavior problems are then conducted. Typically the analyst helps the caregivers to define the target behaviors in terms of what the child does or does not do, or says or does not say. Put differently, the analyst attempts to express the problems through the use of verbs, not adjectives. For example, the informants may initially describe the child as being "hostile" or "lazy." The analyst asks the informants to specify the child's behaviors that suggest those adjectives. Being "hostile" may mean hitting, grabbing, or cursing. Being "lazy" may mean not completing in-seat classroom assignments or home chores. In this way, the analyst determines which behaviors are causing problems.

Exploring Key Parameters

Once the problem behaviors have been defined, the analyst explores their key parameters. The child's parents (or others being interviewed) are guided to estimate each problem's frequency, duration, and intensity. Because most applied behavior analysts believe that behavior is situation-specific, the evaluator is also likely to ask where or under what conditions each behavior occurs. For example, children often behave differently in the presence of strangers than they do in the presence of their parents.

On identifying the setting(s) of the problem behaviors, the analyst then ascertains what environmental conditions precipitate or maintain the behavior. Much effort is spent determining antecedents of the target problem behaviors, that is, those events that typically precede the behaviors. For example, consider a handicapped child who is referred for evaluation because of frequent tantrums during the day. Likely antecedents might include adult requests to complete an educational routine that is difficult for the child and is, therefore, aversive. Through identification of antecedents, the evaluator begins to understand when the problem behaviors are most likely to occur.

A central tenet of the applied behavior approach is that behavior is a function of its consequences. Thus, much attention is also given to delineating those events that follow the occurrence of the target behaviors. As described earlier, many problem behaviors are followed and thus maintained by positive or negative reinforcement. For example, a child's tantrums may be reinforced positively if the caregiver "gives in" and provides the child with what he or she wants. Allowing the child to escape an educational task as a result of tantrums would increase the future probability that tantrums will occur because of negative reinforcement. The applied behavior analyst thoroughly assesses the various caregivers' responses to the child's behavior and, through a consideration of key principles, begins to decipher what functions the problem behaviors serve and what environmental variables maintain them.

Rating Scales and Questionnaires

The evaluator will sometimes employ problem-specific rating scales and questionnaires to elucidate further the caregiver's concerns and to document the presence of a behavior problem. Rating scales are useful tools in the process of diagnosing and classifying specific behavior disorders and are often useful clinically as well. For example, the Conners Teacher Rating Scale (CTRS) (Conners, 1969), reproduced in Figure 2-1 of this textbook, is often used to screen large groups of children for hyperactivity. Use of behavior rating scales can facilitate treatment selection also. A high anxiety factor on the CTRS, for example, may suggest that the use of stimulant medication should be avoided (Barkley, 1981).

Direct Observations

As has been shown, applied behavior analysts often employ structured interviews, checklists, and questionnaires to identify and understand problem behaviors. Their own observations of the child as he or she interacts with others, however, are among behavior analysts' most important tools. The analyst observes the antecedents and consequences of problem behaviors, thus adding to his or her understanding of the problem. After collecting data in these several ways, the analyst then moves to the selection of treatments.

Selection of Treatment Option

At the conclusion of the initial assessment, the applied behavior analyst advises the child's parents (or other caregivers) and, when appropriate, the child whether or not treatment is warranted. If intervention is indicated, the analyst works with the caregiver(s) to develop treatment goals and objectives. Alternative levels of service are then described. These levels range from referral to another professional, with or without written recommendations, to active, ongoing involvement in short-term (8 to 16 sessions) therapy with an emphasis on parent education and training and teacher consultation. If the caregivers elect to participate in treatment, therapist and consumer responsibilities are discussed and are often summarized in a written contract.

Establishing Priorities for Treatment

The order in which specific problem behaviors are treated is determined by the clinician in conjunction with the caregivers. Factors often considered prior to initiation of the therapeutic plan are the availability of effective treatments for the respective high-priority target behaviors, the relative severity of each presenting problem, the degree of effort and sophistication required of the consumers to manage each behavior, consumer preferences, and the professional competencies of the therapist. Behaviors that can be modified solely through positive reinforcement and other basic interventions, or dangerous behaviors that require immediate attention, often are targeted for treatment first. Interventions for behaviors that are not dangerous but that are difficult to alter, such as self-stimulatory behavior, often are delayed until the caregivers have experienced some success in implementing basic strategies directed at more malleable behaviors.

Ongoing Measurement

Assessment continues throughout all phases of treatment. Not only does the therapist assess progress, but also, whenever possible, he or she trains the caregivers and sometimes the child to record their observations of target behaviors as treatment proceeds. Several observation systems have been shown to yield valid measures of clinical gains. These systems are reviewed in detail by Cone and Hawkins (1977), Gelfand and Hartmann (1975), Hersen and Bellack (1976), Mash and Terdal (1981), Ollendick and Hersen (1984), and Sulzer-Azaroff and Mayer (1977).

BEHAVIOR TREATMENT

Enrollment of Caregivers

The handicapped child's primary caregivers, be they parents, teachers, or professional staff, often are in the best position to implement a behavior change program. Already quite experienced with the types of management strategies that are effective with the particular child, they often have established a positive relationship with him or her. They have served as the child's instructors in many situations and are with the child for extended periods, allowing them to conduct multiple learning trials (treatment sessions) on a daily basis. There are also fewer difficulties in generalizing treatment gains to the natural environment (home, school, community) when caregivers serve as the primary behavior change agents.

Enrollment of caregivers can often be difficult, however. Their beliefs and attitudes as well as their other responsibilities may prevent their effective involvement in behavior modification programs. For example, some caregivers may prefer to withdraw because of the child's misbehavior. Others may consider the establishment of contingencies to be overly harsh. Many lay persons (and professionals, too) have misconceptions regarding the principles that govern children's behavior. For example, some mistakenly believe that children should and will behave appropriately in the absence of adult attention, affection, and praise. On the other hand, many caregivers agree with the philosophy of applied behavior analysis but cannot or will not carry out recommended treatment procedures accurately or consistently. Unfortunately, most recommended procedures are time-consuming and repetitious, and require considerable effort if they are to be successful.

Setting the Stage

The clinician begins by establishing an atmosphere that is conducive to learning and cooperation. This is accomplished as the clinician gets acquainted with the child and shows himself or herself to be a friendly, rewarding person. The therapy situation must be seen as nonthreatening. The clinician then provides an overview of the strategies that have been selected to attain the agreed upon treatment goals and solicits input from the clients.

Identifying Reinforcers

The next step entails identifying reinforcers for the child to promote the desired behaviors. Through observations, the therapist works to identify the reinforcers maintaining the troublesome behaviors so that the environment can be altered. These reinforcers are then provided only when some lower rate appropriate behaviors occur. For example, if the child's disruptive behavior (such as interrupting adult conversations or loud and perseverative vocalizations) is being reinforced by the parents' attention, the clinician trains the parents to attend instead to the child's appropriate behavior, that is, to catch the child being "good."

Another method of identifying the child's reinforcers involves observing the child at free play to identify his or her favorite activities. The child's caregivers can also suggest reinforcers, and, when feasible, the verbal child can be asked about his or her reinforcers. With profoundly or severely mentally retarded children who do not engage in spontaneous play or who are nonverbal, systematic presentation of an array of stimuli selected across various sensory channels may be required (Pace, Ivancic, Edwards, Iwata and Page, 1985).

Characteristics of a Useful Reinforcer

As described earlier, a wide variety of verbal statements, activities, manipulable objects, and edible objects are available for use as reinforcers. When selecting among these options, it is important to consider several characteristics of an effective reinforcer.

■ First, the reinforcer should be dispensed immediately following the occurrence of the desirable behavior. In general, immediate reinforcement is more effective than delayed reinforcement because the handicapped child can more easily identify which behaviors result in reinforcement and which do not. This is especially important at the beginning of treatment programs for the disabled.

■ Second, the administration of the reinforcer should be placed exclusively under the caregiver's control, such that the child will gain access to the reinforcer *if and only if* the desired behavior occurs. This is not to suggest that the child is denied his or her usual reinforcers for the duration of treatment. Rather, when possible, extra reinforcers over and above those that the child customarily receives should be chosen. For example, every child is entitled to three meals per day irrespective of his or her behavior. However, it is both ethical and effective to give the child a choice of special snacks or desserts contingent on appropriate behavior.

■ Third, the reinforcer should be dispensed in small amounts. Ideally, reinforcement should be given frequently and in low doses. For example, it is better to distribute a contingent allowance of one quarter on several occasions each day than to award $10 at the end of a successful week.

■ Fourth, the reinforcers should be resistant to satiation. Satiation is a reduction in the patient's performance because of a loss of reinforcer effectiveness. This often occurs after a sizeable amount of a specific reinforcer has been provided within a short time period. All have heard the saying, "Let's not make it too much of a good thing." Particularly when working with the disabled, it is frequently necessary to conduct multiple learning trials designed to promote one behavior and discourage another. Across numerous trials, it is highly probable that the reinforcers will lose their value if dispensed repeatedly. To combat satiation, applied behavior analysts commonly offer a variety of contingent reinforcers, conduct brief training trials that do not result in the distribution of large amounts of reinforcement at any one time, and often rely on conditioned generalized reinforcers, such as verbal approval, points, tokens, and money to promote behavior change.

■ Fifth, the reinforcers should be compatible with the goals of the treatment program. For instance, an obese patient would not be given candy, and a withdrawn child would not be allowed to earn long periods of time alone in his or her room. Furthermore, the reinforcers should be inexpensive, readily available to the caregivers yet accessible to the patient only in limited supply, easily dispensable, easily transportable, relatively novel to the child, and without negative side effects.

Selection of reinforcers is a critical step in the design of all behavior management programs. Once reinforcers have been identified and obtained, providing them usually is contingent on the occurrence of adaptive behavior. Disabled youngsters who are learning new behaviors, however, often require more than contingent reinforcement. It is frequently necessary for the caregiver to provide instruction as well. For example, consider a handicapped youngster who is learning to swallow capsules to comply with a prescribed medication regimen. If the caregivers are only using contingent reinforcement, they may wait a long time for the client to pick up and swallow a capsule so they can provide reinforcement. This obviously would be an extraordinarily inefficient approach to training. Thus, the behavior analyst sometimes must also provide instruction for the clients to develop and change behavior.

Competency-Based Training

To expedite the learning process, the applied behavior analyst may implement a training program that emphasizes both the acquisition and the maintenance of skills. These programs are called competency-based because they are concerned with promoting competent behaviors and skills. The key features of a competency-based training model include the following:

1. Identification of target skills.
2. Analyses of target skills with corresponding operational definitions and assessment instruments.
3. Identification of the student's proficiency in targeted skill areas
   before training.
4. Specification of the learner's objectives.
5. Provision of systematic training through verbal description and
   modeling and completion of behavior rehearsals.
6. Repeated measurement of the child's performance during and
   after training.
7. When necessary, provision of remedial training.

This sequence is illustrated in the following case history.

At the time of referral, Sandy was 17 years old. She was profoundly
mentally retarded. She was diagnosed as having an ornithine
transferase deficiency, an inborn error of metabolism that results
in an accumulation of ammonia as a by-product of protein metabolism. Treatment consisted of a protein-restricted diet combined with
citrulline and phenylbutyrate. Sandy typically accepted the
citrulline when it was placed in a preferred food such as banana
pudding. Because of the extremely bitter taste of phenylbutyrate,
however, she refused to swallow this substance, even when it was
mixed into sweet suspensions, such as chocolate ice cream. The
attending physician reasoned that Sandy would be more likely to
take the phenylbutyrate if it were placed in tasteless gelatin capsules. Unfortunately, Sandy had never taken medication via
capsule. The physician asked the applied behavior analyst to teach
Sandy to swallow 42 large capsules per day.

The behavior analyst began by analyzing the required target
behaviors; that is, she delineated the steps Sandy had to complete
after being given a capsule. Successful capsule-swallowing consists
of the following steps: grasping the capsule by the thumb and index
finger of the dominant hand, opening the mouth, extending the
tongue, placing the capsule toward the back of the tongue, taking
a sip of water, tilting the head back slightly, and swallowing. Prior
to training, Sandy was consistently unable to swallow the capsules.

Treatment began by explaining to Sandy the advantages of
learning to swallow capsules, particularly the fact that she would
no longer need to take her unpleasant-tasting medication in food.
She was also informed that she could earn a star for a chart posted
in her room each time she swallowed a practice candy or capsule
and that stars were exchangeable immediately for preferred
activities, such as singing songs, for grooming aids, such as eye
makeup and lipstick, and treats, such as fruit juice. Training

sessions were conducted twice daily and each consisted of at least ten practice trials. A trial involved handing Sandy a capsule, asking her to swallow it, and recording whether the capsule was accepted or expelled.

At the beginning of each session, the clinician described the steps of successful swallowing and demonstrated the necessary skills. Consistent with the method of shaping successive approximations to the target behavior (described earlier), training materials (candies and capsules) were presented in an order of increasing size. Oblong and spherical cake decoration sprinkles, button-dot and Tic-Tac candies, and progressively larger capsules, first containing corn starch and then phenylbutyrate, were presented in sequence across sessions.

On presentation of each capsule, the clinician used a syringe to squirt 60 ml of water into Sandy's mouth and asked her to swallow the capsule without chewing it. If she chewed the capsule, she was asked to surrender it. On such occasions, she did not earn stars. If Sandy swallowed the capsule without chewing, the clinician would indicate his or her approval through smiles, praise, and hugs. Sandy was then awarded a star and allowed to select her reinforcer. Through employment of repeated instruction, performance-based feedback and contingent reinforcement, Sandy gradually learned to swallow candies and capsules. By the fortieth session, she could consistently swallow 42 large capsules per day.

Sandy's case is an example of a successful competency-based training program whereby a handicapped adolescent learned the desired pill-taking behaviors through systematic instruction and positive reinforcement.

Establishing Alternatives to Misbehavior

Unfortunately, an emphasis on the acquisition of desirable behaviors is not always sufficient. Often the handicapped youngster has multiple problem behaviors that impede educational or medical progress and which, therefore, must be suppressed. When faced with the task of reducing inappropriate behaviors, the applied behavior analyst often begins with reinforcement-centered approaches. Included among these reinforcement-centered approaches are differential reinforcement of other behavior (DRO), differential reinforcement of incompatible behavior (DRI), and differential reinforcement of appropriate behavior (DRA).

Each of these strategies is designed to establish alternative appropriate behaviors while managing or eliminating problem behaviors. For example, using a DRO procedure, an autistic child may receive an edible reward paired with praise every 30 minutes if he or she does not exhibit disruptive behaviors during that half hour. If disruptive behaviors occur, food and praise are withheld until 30 minutes pass without disruption. To illustrate the use of a DRI procedure, consider a blind, severely mentally retarded youth who repeatedly engages in self-injurious behavior, such as eye-poking. Through a DRI program, the applied behavior analyst may provide music contingent on the youth's hand(s) contacting some educational materials such as blocks or clay, a behavior that is incompatible with eye-poking.

Of these three reinforcement-based approaches to establishing acceptable alternatives to misbehavior, differential reinforcement of an appropriate behavior (DRA) is perhaps best because it aims to increase a specific adaptive behavior. For instance, children often are aggressive as they attempt to escape from adult demands. Using a DRA strategy, it is possible that reinforcement of appropriate behavior, such as compliance with adult requests, is sufficient to reduce or eliminate such aggression (Slifer, Ivancic, Parrish, Page, and Burgio, 1986).

Punishment

Reinforcement-centered approaches, however, are not always effective. It may not be possible to identify the reinforcers maintaining the child's misbehaviors and to alter their availability so as to strengthen alternative behaviors. On occasion it may be necessary to add punishment contingencies. Because such procedures can be overused or abused, they should be employed only after reinforcement-based strategies have been shown to be ineffective. Throughout the application of punishment, the therapist must remain sensitive to the rights and welfare of the handicapped child.

Negative Verbal Statement

As indicated earlier, punishment typically involves either the presentation of an unpleasant event or the removal of reinforcers. With respect to the former, for example, the caregiver may issue a *negative verbal statement* in the form of a reprimand or warning following a child's misbehavior. Although often employed during everyday interactions, such negative statements have inconsistent effects. Sometimes they suppress misbehaviors immediately; at other times they serve as reinforcers. The manner in which verbal disapprovals are stated may determine their effectiveness. For instance, in a classroom setting, private reprimands that are delivered softly have been shown to be more effective than loud reprimands that are shouted (O'Leary, Kaufman, Kass, and Drabman,

1970). Verbal punishment is advantageous in that it attempts to manage the handicapped patient's behavior without producing physical discomfort. Drawbacks include the aforementioned inconsistent effects. Often, for example, verbal disapproval makes little difference. Also, because caregivers already rely extensively on verbal punishment, an increase in this practice may be questionable.

Time Out

A strategy that involves the removal of the child from his or her reinforcers is that of *time out*. During the time out interval, the handicapped child does not have access to any of the reinforcers she or he normally enjoys. A variety of time out procedures have been used effectively, including brief physical isolation (Lahey, McNees, and McNees, 1973), partial removal from preferred activities (Porterfield, Herbert-Jackson, and Risley, 1976), and passively precluding the child's opportunities to receive reinforcement (Foxx and Shapiro, 1978; Mansdorf, 1977).

Effective use of time out hinges on several considerations.

■ First, all reinforcers that support the problem behavior must be removed. In homes, time outs often are spent in areas such as hallways or bathrooms, where none of the child's preferred activities take place. At school, time outs are often located in visually shielded corners of the classroom. During time out, all reinforcers should be beyond reach and out of sight.

■ Second, time out will be effective only if the child has been removed from reinforcement; it will not work if he or she has simply been removed from the aversive situation. A mistaken use of time out occurs when teachers remove children from classrooms because of misbehavior, assuming that such disciplinary removals constitute time out. These removals, however, may actually result in increases in disruptive behaviors if the child is escaping from an aversive academic assignment. If this occurs, the problem behavior has inadvertently been reinforced negatively.

■ Third, with some handicapped youngsters the use of time out may be ill advised. Among children for whom time out may be unsuitable are those who are self-stimulatory, socially withdrawn, or combative. Many handicapped children engage in self-stimulatory behaviors, such as body rocking, daydreaming, or masturbation. If placed in a relatively barren, isolated, nonstimulating area, the patient is likely to turn to self-stimulatory behaviors, thereby defeating the purpose of time out. In addition, isolation from others may be undesirable for children who lack social skills. For these children, time out may serve only to further isolate them at a time when the development of social behaviors should be the focus of treatment. Neither is time out a sensible alternative when patients are so resistant or combative that they cannot be positioned or maintained in the time out area.

■ Fourth, time out should be administered as consistently as possible. Especially at the beginning of a treatment program, time out should be implemented every time the targeted problem behavior occurs. Time out should not be directed intermittently at a number of problem behaviors.

■ Fifth, the duration of time out should be kept short. Brief time outs are often effective in suppressing misbehavior, whereas long time outs can sometimes be counterproductive (White, Nielson, and Johnson, 1972).

■ Sixth, shaping the child's engagement in a desirable alternative behavior along with the time out enhances the effectiveness of time out. For example, if students are permitted to converse with one another during scheduled periods of unstructured activity each day, a time out contingent on talking out of turn during structured classroom activities is more likely to be effective.

■ A final consideration: time out should be employed sparingly. Because it consists of the removal of the child from reinforcement, those caregivers who implement it are likely to be resented by the child. Consequently, the child may work to avoid such caregivers or may actually strike out against them. Most clinicians and educators are concerned primarily with helping the child acquire skills and, therefore, they use time out only when misbehaviors interfere significantly with the child's learning.

Response Cost

Another common method of punishment involving the removal of reinforcement is that of *response cost*. Response cost entails the loss of a positive reinforcer or the imposition of a penalty when the child misbehaves (Kazdin, 1984). With children, response cost usually involves removal of a privilege or part of an allowance. To implement a response-cost contingency, the child must be receiving positive reinforcement that can be withdrawn if he or she misbehaves. The precise fine associated with each type of misbehavior is determined in advance and applied consistently.

Response cost is frequently employed through token economies or point systems within which reinforcement is dispensed for appropriate behaviors and taken away for infractions. To use response cost effectively, it is often necessary to permit the handicapped patient to accumulate a reserve of reinforcers (tokens, points) and cash them in frequently for privileges. Response cost has its largest impact after a patient has had an opportunity to spend the available currency. The patient is then more eager to avoid loss of points or tokens. Small fines are sometimes very effective; with patients who have a history of heavy fines, however, slight penalties may not be enough.

Whenever possible, it is important to inform patients that particular accomplishments will result in positive reinforcement and that certain misbehaviors will lead to fines. As with other punishment techniques, response cost strategies may generate avoidance or aggressive behaviors toward the responsible caregivers. In general, however, response cost is relatively easy to implement, especially when employed with positive reinforcement procedures. There is much evidence to suggest that response cost often produces powerful and rapid reductions in problem behaviors, with possible long-lasting effects.

Overcorrection

Another punishment procedure that involves a penalty for engaging in undesirable behavior is *overcorrection*. This strategy consists of two components. The first component, often termed restitution, pertains to correcting the damages caused by the inappropriate behavior. The second component, positive practice, requires the handicapped child to repeatedly practice an acceptable alternative behavior. For example, consider a disabled child who steals a soft drink from a store. On discovery of the theft, the child is escorted back to the store, where he or she is prompted to return the stolen drink or pay for it, apologizing to the proprietor. This is the restitution component. The child is then encouraged to select additional items and to purchase them with his or her own money. This is the positive practice component.

Overcorrection is frequently employed with handicapped children who are learning independent toileting skills. When an accident occurs, the child is guided to correct the accident (remove and replace wet clothes and bed linens) and to practice going to the bathroom. Overcorrection might also be used when, for example, a preschooler purposefully dumps a glass of milk on the kitchen floor. The child would be given a wet washcloth to sponge up the milk. Once the cloth is rinsed, the child is instructed to use it to scrub a much larger area of the kitchen floor.

If overcorrection is to be successful in changing problem behaviors, it is important that both the restitution and positive practice components be directly related to the problem behavior. It is also important that restitution and positive practice be applied immediately and without pause and that the child have no access to reinforcement throughout the overcorrection procedure. Overcorrection has several advantages.

First, it promotes learning of adaptive skills. The positive practice component is designed to teach appropriate behaviors, a function not inherent in other punishment strategies. Also, overcorrection is less likely than intense punishment to engender withdrawal, aggression, or negative self-statements. It does not induce pain or model aggressive behavior, and its effects are often rapid and long-lasting.

A few difficulties may arise during implementation of the overcorrection procedure. Many children may be unwilling to complete the tasks that constitute the restitution and positive practice sequence. If substantial physical force is necessary to guide a resistant child through the procedure, another disciplinary strategy should be considered. Overcorrection often requires more supervision than alternative punishments. At least one caregiver is needed to monitor the child's progress, and in some settings it may not be possible for staff members to provide such one-to-one supervision.

Negative verbal statements, time out from reinforcement, response cost, and overcorrection are among the most widely used punishment techniques. Several other strategies have been used with handicapped children, including spanking; contingent lemon juice, aromatic ammonia, water mist; contingent protective equipment and restraints; electric shock; contingent exercise; and stimulus satiation. These alternative punishment procedures are not described here because they can be especially aversive, intrusive, and restrictive. Their specific uses require careful scrutiny and the approval of human rights committees.

Considerations when Using Punishment

The use of punishment of any sort is very controversial. Generally, punishment should not be introduced until reinforcement strategies have failed to change a child's behavior. If punishment is used, extreme care must be taken to review the rationale for it with the child's guardians and, when possible, with the child himself or herself. They should also be told of potential negative side effects of punishment such as aggression toward the punishing caregiver and the possible suppression of behaviors other than the one targeted for change.

Factors Influencing Effectiveness of Punishment

Once the guardians comprehend the pros and cons of using punishment, their consent is sought. If it is obtained, the selected punishment procedure is applied. The effectiveness of the chosen punishment is a function of several variables: its immediacy and intensity, its schedule of occurrence, the availability from others of reinforcement for the punished response, the timing of punishment in the chain of events leading to the target problem behavior, and the delivery of reinforcement for alternative, appropriate behaviors.

When administering a punishment program, it is important to adhere to the following guidelines:

1. Be sure that the child cannot escape a warranted punishment. The punishment is not likely to be effective if, for example, the child can ignore verbal reprimands, can play with a favorite toy during time out, can go outside rather than complete an over-correction procedure, or can talk his or her way out of a response cost.

2. Make punishment as intense as possible, as long as it does not cause physical injury. In general, the higher the intensity of the aversive event, the greater the response suppression. Punishment is more effective if it is first applied at full intensity than if its intensity is increased gradually. For example, a firm but matter-of-fact ''no'' is superior to an apologetic request to stop, which is followed by louder and louder reprimands. This guideline, however, does not serve as a justification for extended time outs or excessively large fines.

3. Apply punishment every time the target behavior occurs. Punishment is more effective when the negative consequence is delivered consistently rather than every once in a while.

4. Apply punishment immediately following the misbehavior. In this way, the handicapped child is more likely to understand what behavior is being punished.

5. Eliminate any reinforcement that maintains the problem behavior. Parents and teachers often reinforce the very inappropriate behaviors they hope to decrease. For example, when the child has been aggressive, they may scold, issue threats, or lecture as they are revoking a privilege. At the time that discipline is warranted, it would be far better if the parents withheld their attention as much as possible and instead simply stated the contingency and then enforced it (''You hit your brother; go to time out'').

6. Be careful that the delivery of punishment is not associated with the delivery of reinforcement. For instance, parents are often overwhelmed with guilt after spanking their child for misbehaving. They then shower the child with affection and reassurances of their love. In so doing, the child may learn that punishment precedes reinforcement, and he or she may increase the misbehavior.

7. Avoid prolonged or extensive use of punishment. As with reinforcement, if it is used too much or too often, punishment loses
its effectiveness.

8. Provide punishment early in the child's approach toward a
targeted undesirable behavior. Frequently a problem behavior
does not occur in isolation but as part of a sequence of behaviors.
For example, a self-injurious behavior associated with an adult
request to complete an academic task may be preceded by noncompliance, object throwing, tantrums, or aggression. Punishment for the earlier noncompliance may reduce self-injurious
behavior to a greater extent than punishment after the self-
injurious behavior has occurred. It is wiser to punish the child
when she or he reaches for a match than after the fire has been
set.

When to Use Punishment

Because of its possible negative side effects and the ethical considerations cited earlier, punishment procedures should be
implemented infrequently and cautiously. Reinforcement strategies
typically should be attempted first. As already indicated, suppression
of a behavior does not always require punishment. There are situations
in which punishment will be necessary, however. Use of punishment
is defensible when the inappropriate behavior is dangerous to the
handicapped youngster or to others. Under such circumstances,
immediate suppression of the dangerous behavior is necessary. In such
a situation, caregivers cannot wait until the delayed effects of reinforcement and planned ignoring take over.

Punishment is most effective when it is combined with reinforcement. Typically, punishment will only reduce inappropriate behaviors;
it does nothing to teach the child acceptable behaviors. Teaching
children how to behave in socially acceptable ways almost always
requires the use of reinforcement procedures.

WORKING WITH PARENTS AND TEACHERS

Methods of Promoting Generalization

In the previous sections an overview of basic principles and
methods of applied behavior analysis and how they can be used on
behalf of handicapped children and youth was provided. As noted
earlier, behavior occurs in specific situations. A behavior that is reinforced repeatedly in one particular set of circumstances is likely to recur

in that situation. It may also occur in other, similar situations. If a behavior that is reinforced in one setting also increases in other settings (although it is not reinforced in these other settings), *stimulus generalization* is said to have occurred. Examples of such transfers of behavior to different situations are common in everyday life. For instance, if a handicapped youth has learned to use a coin-operated washing machine in a sheltered workshop setting, he or she may be able to use a washer located in a nearby laundromat if the two machines are similar.

Generalization occurs not only across situations but also across behaviors. Changing one behavior may influence other behaviors. For example, reinforcement of instruction-following may also result in decreases in aggression, disruption, and property destruction (Parrish, Cataldo, Kolko, Neef, and Egel, 1986; Russo, Cataldo, and Cushing, 1981). The reinforcement of a behavior may increase the frequency of behaviors that are similar in form or function. This is called *response generalization*.

Applied behavior analysts, like other clinicians, typically assess and treat specific target behaviors in specific settings. For instance, the behavior analyst may respond to a request by a concerned parent, teacher, or physician to diagnose and modify an inappropriate behavior in a particular setting. The treatment strategies outlined earlier often result in marked improvements in the behavior of handicapped children in the settings in which the treatment contingencies are applied. Such accomplishments are relatively insignificant, however, if treatment effects do not last or do not carry over to new situations and behaviors. Unfortunately, the impact of treatment often is highly specific and short-lived.

Behavior analysts have developed numerous strategies for ensuring that clinical gains "maintain" or extend over time and "generalize" or "transfer" across situations and behaviors (Stokes and Baer, 1977). Analysts program for maintenance and generalization rather than assume that treatment effects will endure and be transferred. One of the common strategies employed by behavior analysts to promote maintenance and generalization is sequential modification. If desired behaviors have not transferred to other settings or behaviors as hoped, specific steps are taken to introduce contingency management programs (reinforcement, extinction, or punishment procedures) to each of the behaviors or settings in which transfer is insufficient. For example, consider the case of a child diagnosed as having learning disabilities. An intervention to improve the child's poor academic performance has been shown to be effective in only two of six subject areas. In this circumstance, the intervention may be modified and introduced into each of the four problem areas one after another. Treatment continues until the child's academic performance is adequate across all subjects. The practice of many behavior analysts is characterized by the use of sequential modification.

Another strategy that is used to help maintain and transfer behavior is bringing behavior under the control of consequences that naturally occur in everyday life. When employing this strategy, the analyst tries to set "behavior traps." That is, once a handicapped child's behavior is shaped appropriately, it becomes "trapped" into the system of reinforcers available daily. For example, a teacher might modify the low rate at which a child initiates play with peers through the use of praise and tokens. As the child learns to initiate play, the reinforcers inherent to cooperative play may be sufficient to maintain the acquired social skills, and the teacher's praise and the tokens can be faded out gradually.

Presenting multiple exemplars during training is another method of enhancing maintenance and generalization. This involves providing the handicapped youngster with many opportunities to see and practice learned skills across slightly different situations. For example, if the goal is to teach a developmentally delayed youth to operate a cash register, he or she is given several opportunities to accept money and return correct change. The clinician presents various bills and coins and instructs the youth how to carry out many different transactions. Each type of problem is presented several times until the young person demonstrates a generalized ability to provide correct change.

Maintenance and generalization can also be promoted through training loosely, that is, teaching a behavior imprecisely in settings that are not highly controlled. To illustrate, consider the disabled child who has an overly protective parent who always tells the child exactly how to dress for school. In this situation, the child has become quite dependent on the parent's instructions. When the parent is available to provide guidance, the child wears clothing suitable in terms of warmth, water resistance, color, style, and expense. When the parent is absent, however, the child flounders because he or she has not learned to select proper clothing independently. Through training loosely, the parent sometimes gives the child the opportunity to choose what to wear, sometimes comments about the child's selection, sometimes advises the child about what to wear, sometimes tells the child what to wear, and sometimes says absolutely nothing, leaving it up to the child's teachers or peers to offer feedback. In this way, the child is more likely to acquire "good taste" with respect to clothing.

Use of indiscriminable contingencies can also promote maintenance and generalization. In this situation, the reinforcement or punishment contingencies are arranged so that the handicapped child cannot tell for sure whether or not contingencies are in effect and, consequently, behaves appropriately across situations in hopes of receiving reinforcement and avoiding punishment An example of this is a teacher who attempts to modify three inappropriate behaviors (talking out of turn, getting out of a chair without permission, and using foul language) by sometimes putting contingencies in effect for only one of these behaviors, with the students not knowing which one. The teacher does this by keeping a daily frequency count of one of the three behaviors. At the end of the school day, the teacher provides reinforcement to the students if the frequency of the selected behavior is below a certain number.

Another way to promote maintenance and transfer of desirable behavior is to train with the same materials and under the same conditions that the child will encounter in his or her natural environment. This is known as programming common stimuli. For instance, when preparing a handicapped youth for participation in a sheltered workshop, it would maximize transfer if the training tasks and supplies were similar to those that will be encountered in the sheltered workshop. If the youth were about to accept a position requiring him or her to disassemble four carburetors an hour independently, training should center on carburetor disassembly at faster and faster rates for longer and longer periods under conditions simulating the workshop.

Language and self-management procedures often serve as mediators between initial training and the generalization of learning to new settings and behaviors. Competent performance is not as likely to be restricted to a single setting or behavior if handicapped youngsters can be trained to control their own behavior. If youngsters can learn to deliver reinforcing or punishing consequences to themselves, their behavior is more likely to be maintained. Research has shown that many handicapped clients can monitor their own behavior, establish performance criteria for reinforcement, and determine the amount of reinforcement that they have earned. For example, an impulsive child might be taught to use self-instruction combined with self-reinforcement to reduce his or her rate of careless errors when completing mathematics assignments. If successful, this self-management program could be transferred to other academic subject areas in which impulsivity is a problem.

When training is concluding, gradual removal (fading) of the contingencies is less noticeable to most youngsters than abrupt removal and increases the likelihood that progress will be maintained. Abrupt withdrawal of reinforcing and punishing consequences may result in loss of treatment gains. Gradual withdrawal of contingencies can be accomplished in many ways. For instance, suppose a handicapped child receives five tokens every time he or she washes the supper dishes. To enhance maintenance, the caregiver gradually decreases the number of tokens awarded for each occurrence of dishwashing and on some days simply expresses appreciation for work well done.

Gradual withdrawal of contingencies may be especially helpful because it prepares the client for the "real world." In everyday life, contingencies frequently are not systematic and differential consequences are delayed, if they are provided at all. As was stated earlier, when a behavior is first being acquired or punished, it is essential that consequences be provided immediately and consistently. Once the desired behavior change has occurred, however, its maintenance can be enhanced if consequences are gradually delayed and presented intermittently. For example, a previously reinforced behavior is more resistant to extinction following an intermittent schedule of reinforcement. Once a skill is in a handicapped child's repertoire, it is best to acknowledge it every so often rather than every time it occurs.

Clients can also be trained "to generalize," that is, instructed to demonstrate a learned behavior in different forms and settings and at different times. Parents often do this with their children, asking them, for example, to make another object with blocks or draw another picture with their crayons. Teachers do this as well when they ask for additional answers to a posed question.

These methods of facilitating maintenance and generalization are not mutually exclusive. They can be employed either in isolation or in combination with one another. Especially when working with handicapped clients, it is probable that several of these procedures will have to be used to achieve maintenance and generalization.

Parent Training

The methods of behavior change discussed earlier were developed for use by applied behavior analysts. Behavior analysts have long contended, however, that their methods can have more far-reaching effects if they are employed by a child's parents or teachers. Thus, behavior analysts have developed numerous parent training packages to help parents manage the behavior problems of their children and facilitate the transfer of learned behaviors from the clinic to the home.

Parent training procedures range from informal tips extended to parents on the telephone to intensive parent training programs. Less structured forms of parent training include "how to" books on behavior management, articles on positive parenting found in popular magazines, lectures and workshops by private practitioners and allied professionals, and replies to questions during talk show broadcasts. Numerous highly structured parent training programs are also available.

Intensive parent training programs generally are presented after an initial evaluation of the handicapped child's behavior. Most parent training programs begin with the therapist's describing the contingency management procedures that the parent will carry out in the home and giving a rationale for each of the procedures selected. The therapist encourages the parent to ask questions and to summarize the therapist's directions to assess whether the parents understand who is to do what when.

A modeling component may be included in parent training programs whereby the recommended treatment procedures are demonstrated either through applications with the child, role playing, or videotaped vignettes. The parent is then asked to rehearse the demonstrated behaviors. This typically involves role playing with the therapist portraying the child and the parent rehearsing the application of the procedures. This is done to give the parent practice in a controlled situation in which the therapist can dictate the various situations that may arise at home, and to provide feedback to the parent about his or her performance. Once the parent has demonstrated skill mastery during the role plays, the therapist may have the parent implement the recommended strategies with the child.

Behavior analysts often give the parents a brief written protocol that is procedure or problem specific. These protocols serve as summaries of "do's" and "don'ts." Sessions frequently conclude with homework assignments that require the parent to observe and record the occurrence of target behaviors, to implement prescribed interventions, and to complete relevant reading.

Thereafter, the behavior analyst and the parent will engage in "troubleshooting." When the parents have implemented the procedures at home for a time (perhaps 1 to 2 weeks), they return to the therapist with the data collected on the target behaviors. The therapist reviews the data with the parents and then modifies the procedures and gives further instruction if necessary.

Parent training programs cover a wide range of problem behaviors for which a variety of effective treatment protocols have been developed. Some of these behavior problems include enuresis; encopresis; hyperactivity; parental, medical, or educational noncompliance; lying; stealing; verbal abuse; fire-setting; property destruction; disruptive behaviors; self-injury; feeding problems; obesity; tantrums; pica; inappropriate sexual behaviors; phobias; and lack of social skills. For reviews of the extensive literature on behavioral approaches to parent education, the reader is referred to Berkowitz and Graziano (1972), Dangel and Polster (1984), Forehand and Atkeson (1977), Graziano (1977), Johnson and Katz (1973), McMahon and Forehand (1980), Moreland, Schwebel, Beck, and Wells (1982), and O'Dell (1974).

Teacher Consultation

Behavioral approaches to assessment and treatment are used widely by special educators to manage a variety of behavior and learning difficulties. Applied behavior analysts frequently provide consultation to teachers. The consultative process begins when contact is first made between the therapist and teacher. It is important to note that when the school-related contact is made, the teacher should be the first to be contacted, rather than other administrative personnel. If a teacher feels slighted by other personnel being contacted before him or her, the consultative relationship may be adversely affected. After discussing the child's problem behaviors, the applied behavior analyst will schedule a school visit if it is requested.

During the school visit, the behavior analyst conducts a semistructured interview, like that described earlier, and may ask the teacher to respond to rating scales or questionnaires. Together the behavior analyst and teacher identify, define, and examine the key parameters of behaviors to be targeted for change, often observing and recording the target behaviors to obtain objective baseline measures of the problem behaviors. The analyst devises a measurement system that can be adapted to the teacher's schedule and that is sufficiently precise to evaluate treatment effects. The analyst may visit the classroom periodically to help the teacher obtain valid and reliable data.

Once a baseline has been established, the behavior analyst will design a contingency management program with the teacher and will model the intervention procedures. As with parents, the behavior analyst will also encourage the teacher to rehearse the chosen procedures. Several factors are considered when developing a treatment procedure. Previous research has shown that behavioral interventions that are designed to increase appropriate behavior and that require little time to implement are rated more acceptable to teachers (Reimers, Wacker, and Koeppl, 1987). Thus, the use of treatment procedures with these characteristics may help to promote teacher compliance with recommendations. The following case history shows how analyst, teacher, and parent worked together to improve a child's behavior.

Bill was a $6\frac{1}{2}$-year-old boy referred by his pediatrician to an outpatient clinic specializing in child behavior management. He was referred because of his reported disruptiveness, hyperactivity, short attention span, and poor academic performance. He was accompanied by his mother to the behavior management clinic on the day of the initial evaluation. During the evaluation, he frequently interrupted his mother while she was talking and went quickly from one activity to another.

His teacher was contacted by telephone to get her opinions about Bill's behavior and academic performance. The concerns expressed by Bill's teacher were consistent with those reported by his mother. His short attention span contributed to his not following directions and not staying on-task. His disruptiveness was a concern at school as well as at home. In the classroom, Bill often talked or got out of his seat without permission. At home, Bill often interrupted his mother when she was talking on the telephone or when she was visiting with guests. Bill was also reported to be underachieving academically. According to his teacher, he seldom completed homework assignments.

After the initial evaluation, the therapist met with Bill's mother and teacher to discuss methods of measuring the target behaviors. After the behaviors had been defined operationally, it was agreed that Bill's teacher would record occurrences of disruptive behavior in the classroom. The teacher also agreed to record his daily percentage of compliance with verbal requests, as well as the percentage of homework assignments completed. His mother agreed to record the frequency with which he completed five daily chores and the frequency with which Bill interrupted her when she was either on the telephone or visiting with a guest. She also kept a frequency count of the total number of times she talked on the telephone or visited with a guest to get the percentage of interrupted conversations.

At the end of 1 week of data collection, the therapist met with Bill, his mother, and his teacher to review the data and discuss various treatment options. A home-based token economy was selected as the treatment of choice. The token economy was set up at both the school and the home to provide for generalization of treatment effects across settings. Under this system, Bill was given an opportunity to earn tokens at home and at school for exhibiting certain appropriate behaviors and was allowed to exchange the tokens daily at home for certain reinforcers (toys, soda, extra television viewing time, and trips to the movie theater). Varying point values were assigned to each of the reinforcers. For example, a soda cost fewer tokens than a trip to the movie theater.

The therapist explained the system to Bill, his mother, and his teacher and had each sign a written contract stating their responsibilities. Each received a protocol describing the target appropriate behaviors and the contingent privileges. The therapist then modeled how to administer a token to Bill when he performed an appropriate behavior and gave them an opportunity to rehearse the procedure. The therapist then met separately with Bill and his mother to discuss the procedures for exchanging tokens for reinforcers. It was agreed that Bill would keep a record of his performance on a chart posted on the refrigerator. It was also agreed that the token economy would remain in effect for a period of 2 weeks, at which time it would be reviewed and any necessary modifications made. During this interval, both Bill's teacher and his mother agreed to continue collecting data on the behaviors targeted for change.

At the end of 2 weeks, the therapist met with Bill, his mother, and his teacher to discuss the token economy and to review the data. The data indicated that Bill's behavior had begun to improve in nearly all of the targeted areas. Bill was receiving his tokens for each of the appropriate target behaviors he demonstrated, and he enthusiastically exchanged his tokens daily for his rewards. The only behavior that did not seem to be improving was Bill's interruptions when his mother was with a friend. Thus, it was decided to raise the point value for appropriate behavior during these times. Also, it was decided that a response cost would be added to the system, which involved the loss of a token following any interruption during a friend's visit. The therapist agreed to make weekly phone contacts with both Bill's mother and teacher to monitor his progress and to "troubleshoot" any problems that might arise.

Applied Behavior Analysis and Medicine

The principles and methods of applied behavior analysis are increasingly being used in connection with medical treatment. Behavioral techniques have been shown to be effective in partially ameliorating illnesses as diverse as asthma, cardiovascular disease, chronic pain, urinary and fecal incontinence, obesity, and recurrent abdominal pain. Behavioral medicine has also made significant contributions in the areas of exercise, smoking cessation, preparation for medical and surgical procedures, compliance with therapeutic regimens, and cost containment with respect to health care delivery. Readers interested in learning more about behavioral medicine as it pertains to handicapped youth are encouraged to consult the following sources: Ferguson and Taylor (1980), Krasnegor, Arasteh, and Cataldo (1986), McGrath and Firestone (1983), Russo and Varni (1982), and Varni (1983). The following case history illustrates the relevance of behavioral strategies to the management of a chronic medical disorder.

Seth, an 11-year-old boy diagnosed as having Prader-Willi syndrome, was admitted to an inpatient unit specializing in the treatment of severe behavior disorders. He weighed 61 kg (134 lb) and was 143.5 cm (4 feet 8 inches) tall. He had small hands and feet, abnormal facial features, hypogonadism, and moderate mental retardation. Seth was admitted to the hospital because of overeating, which had resulted in extreme obesity and cardiopulmonary complications. He suffered sleep apnea, a condition in which he stopped breathing for brief periods. He attempted to rest each night while sitting upright in a chair. His mother had installed a lock on the family refrigerator and kept nonrefrigerated food in the trunk of the family car. Despite daily parental efforts to control his food consumption, Seth managed to obtain off-limits food at home, at school, and in the community.

At admission, he was restricted to 1200 calories per day. During inpatient treatment sessions conducted in a room equipped with a one-way mirror and two tables and a chair, Seth was given an opportunity to play in the presence of food. Puzzles, coloring books, crayons, magazines, and scissors were placed on one table. Food items, including small bits of chocolate candy, salted peanuts, potato chips, and cups containing soft drinks, were distributed on the second table.

A series of assessments was conducted prior to treatment during which a therapist accompanied Seth into the training room and encouraged him to interact with the play materials. After Seth had begun playing, the therapist excused herself, saying she had work to do and would return later. The therapist invited Seth to continue doing whatever he desired, but cautioned, "Now remember, it's not snack time, so don't take any food," and left the room. Throughout several assessment sessions, the frequency of food consumption was observed and recorded. Food consumption was defined as any instance of a piece of food coming in contact with Seth's mouth. Repeated bites from the same piece of food were scored as separate episodes of consumption. Seth's baseline rate of food consumption was 2.6 episodes per minute.

After this initial assessment, the clinician employed differential reinforcement to strengthen behaviors other than food consumption (DRO). A DRO procedure using token-mediated reinforcement was implemented. The initial length of the DRO interval was set at 10 seconds. When Seth did not consume food for 10 seconds, the therapist entered the room, delivered praise and gave him tokens. If he had eaten, the therapist entered the room at the end of the interval and informed Seth that he would not get tokens. The therapist then left the room and the next interval was begun.

If Seth had accumulated 10 tokens at the end of the session, he was given an opportunity to trade them for a low-calorie food item or toy of his choice. Available food items consisted of sugarless gum and lollipops, a diet soda, and apples. After three consecutive intervals without food consumption, the interval was doubled—10 seconds, 20 seconds, 40 seconds, and so forth—with the outcome that some treatment sessions were as long as 60 minutes. Implementation of DRO procedures with token reinforcement resulted in an average rate of 0.5 episodes of food consumption during the first treatment session and no food intake during subsequent sessions.

Seth had gained 5.5 kg (12 lb) during the 6-month period prior to admission. During his hospitalization, he lost 1.5 kg (3.3 lb). Follow-up sessions reflected maintenance of decreases in rate of food consumption for 9 weeks after discharge, with accompanying improvements in cardiopulmonary functioning.

This case history demonstrates how applied behavior analysis can be used in the management of a medical disorder. Seth's behavioral changes resulted in improved physical health.

SUMMARY

In this chapter, an attempt was made to provide an introduction to the principles and procedures of applied behavior analysis, a burgeoning area of scientific and clinical activity aimed at the development and use of practical solutions for socially significant problems. These principles and procedures have been derived from extensive experimental research and often are applied quite effectively on behalf of handicapped children and youth. The considerations and steps typically taken by applied behavior analysts when designing assessment and treatment programs for handicapped youngsters have been outlined and illustrated through actual case material. In and of itself, this chapter does not adequately prepare any individual to implement the strategies reviewed herein. It is designed to be more a resource than a recipe. Prior to practicing the described procedures, each interested individual should receive extensive training and arrange for ongoing supervision. Such supervision should be predicated on reliable outcome data that clearly indicate the individual client's response to treatment and should occur in the context of a peer review process that promotes adherence to ethical standards.

REFERENCES

Achenbach, T.M., and Edelbrock, C.S. (1979). The child behavior profile: II. Boys aged 12–16 and girls aged 6–11 and 12–16. *Journal of Consulting and Clinical Psychology, 47*, 223–233.

Alberto, P.A., and Troutman, A.C. (1982). *Applied behavior analysis for teachers: Influencing student performance*. Columbus, Ohio: Charles E. Merrill.

Baer, D.M., Wolf, M.M., and Risley, T.R. (1968). Some current dimensions of applied behavior analysis. *Journal of Applied Behavior Analysis, 1*, 91–97.

Bandura, A. (1969). *Principles of behavior modification*. New York: Holt, Rinehart and Winston.

Bandura, A. (1977). *Social learning theory*. Englewood Cliffs, New Jersey: Prentice-Hall.

Barkley, R.A. (1981). *Hyperactive children: A handbook for diagnosis and treatment*. New York: Guilford Press.

Berkowitz, B.P., and Graziano, A.M. (1972). Training parents as behavior therapists: A review. *Behavior Research and Therapy, 10,* 297–317.

Catania, A.C. (1984). *Learning* (2nd Ed.). Englewood Cliffs, New Jersey: Prentice-Hall.

Cone, J.E., and Hawkins, R.P. (1977). *Behavioral assessment: New directions in clinical psychology.* New York: Brunner/Mazel.

Conners, C.K. (1969). A teacher rating scale for use in drug studies with children. *American Journal of Psychiatry, 126,* 884–888.

Dangel, R.F., and Polster, R.A. (1984). *Parent training: Foundations of research and practice.* New York: Guilford Press.

Eyberg, S.M. (1980). Eyberg Child Behavior Inventory. *Journal of Clinical Child Psychology, 9,* 29.

Ferguson, J.M., and Taylor, C.B. (1980). *The comprehensive handbook of behavioral medicine.* New York: SP Medical and Scientific Books.

Forehand, R.L., and Atkeson, B. (1977). Generalization of treatment effects with parents as therapists: A review of assessment and implementation procedures. *Behavior Therapy, 8,* 575–593.

Foxx, R.M., and Shapiro, S. T. (1978). The time-out ribbon: A nonexclusionary timeout procedure. *Journal of Applied Behavior Analysis, 11,* 125–136.

Gelfand, D.M., and Hartmann, D.P. (1975). *Child behavior analysis and therapy.* New York: Pergamon.

Graziano, A.M. (1977). Parents as behavior therapists. In M. Hersen, R.M. Eisler, and P.M. Miller (Eds.), *Progress in behavior modification (Vol. 4).* New York: Academic Press.

Hersen, M., and Bellack, A.S. (1976). *Behavioral assessment: A practical handbook.* New York: Pergamon Press.

Hilgard, E.R., and Bower, G.H. (1966). *Theories of learning.* (3rd Ed.). New York: Appleton-Century-Crofts.

Honig, W.K., and Staddon, J.E.R. (1977). *Handbook of operant behavior.* Englewood Cliffs, New Jersey: Prentice-Hall.

Johnson, C.A., and Katz, R.C. (1973). Using parents as change agents for their children: A review. *Journal of Child Psychology and Psychiatry, 14,* 181–200.

Kanfer, F.H., and Phillips, J.S. (1970). *Learning foundations of behavior therapy.* New York: John Wiley and Sons.

Kazdin, A.E. (1984). *Behavior modification in applied settings.* Homewood, Illinois: Dorsey Press.

Krasnegor, N.A., Arasteh, J.D., and Cataldo, M.F. (1986). *Child health behavior: A behavioral pediatrics perspective.* New York: John Wiley and Sons.

Lahey, B.B., McNees, P.M., and McNees, M.C. (1973). Control of an obscene "verbal tic" through timeout in an elementary school classroom. *Journal of Applied Behavior Analysis, 6,* 101–104.

Mansdorf, I.J. (1977) Reinforcer isolation: An alternative to subject isolation in time-out from positive reinforcement. *Journal of Behavior Therapy and Experimental Psychiatry, 8,* 391–393.

Mash, E.J., and Terdal, L.G. (1981). *Behavioral assessment of childhood disorders.* New York: Guilford Press.

Matson, J.L. and Mulick, J. (1983). *Handbook of mental retardation.* Elmsford, New York: Pergamon Books.

McGrath, P.J., and Firestone, P. (1983). *Pediatric and adolescent behavioral medicine: Issues in treatment.* New York: Springer Publishing Co.

McMahon, R.J., and Forehand, R.L. (1980). Self-help behavior therapies in parent training. In B.B. Lahey and A. E. Kazdin (Eds), *Advances in clinical child psychology (Vol. 3).* New York: Plenum.

Miller, L.K. (1980). *Principles of everyday behavior analysis.* 2nd Ed. Monterey, CA: Brooks/Cole Publishing Co.

Moreland, J.R., Schwebel, A.I., Beck, S., and Wells, R. (1982). Parents as therapists: A review of the behavior therapy parent training literature—1975 to 1981. *Behavior Modification, 6,* 250-276.

O'Dell, S. (1974). Training parents in behavior modification: A review. *Psychological Bulletin, 81,* 418-433.

O'Leary, K.D., Kaufman, K.F., Kass, R., and Drabman, R. (1970). The effects of loud and soft reprimands on the behavior of disruptive students. *Exceptional Children, 37,* 145-155.

Ollendick, T.H. and Hersen, M. (1984). *Child behavioral assessment: Principles and procedures.* New York: Pergamon.

Pace, G.M., Ivancic, M.T., Edwards, G.L., Iwata, B.A., and Page, T.J. (1985). Assessment of stimulus preference and reinforcer value with profoundly retarded individuals. *Journal of Applied Behavior Analysis, 18,* 249-255.

Parrish, J.M., Cataldo, M.F., Kolko, D.J., Neef, N.A., and Egel, A.L. (1986). Experimental analysis of response covariation among compliant and inappropriate behaviors. *Journal of Applied Behavior Analysis, 19,* 241-254.

Pavlov, I.P. (1927). *Conditioned reflexes.* London: Oxford University Press.

Porterfield, J.K., Herbert-Jackson, E., and Risley, T.R. (1976). Contingent observation: An effective and acceptable procedure for reducing disruptive behavior of young children in a group setting. *Journal of Applied Behavior Analysis, 9,* 55-64.

Quay, H.C., and Peterson, D.R. (1979). *Manual for the behavior problem checklist.* Published by the authors at 59 Fifth St., Highland Park, New Jersey, 08904.

Reimers, T.M., Wacker, D.P., and Koeppl, G. (1987). Acceptability of behavioral interventions: A review of the literature. *School Psychology Review, 16,* 212-227.

Russo, D.C., Cataldo, M.F., and Cushing, P.J. (1981). Compliance training and behavioral covariation in the treatment of multiple behavior problems. *Journal of Applied Behavior Analysis, 14,* 209-222.

Russo, D.C., and Varni, J.W. (1982). *Behavioral pediatrics: Research and practice.* New York: Plenum Press.

Skinner, B.F. (1953). *Science and human behavior.* New York: Macmillan.

Slifer, K.J., Ivancic, M.T., Parrish, J.M., Page, T.J., and Burgio, L.D. (1986). Assessment and treatment of multiple behavior problems exhibited by a profoundly retarded adolescent. *Journal of Behavior Therapy and Experimental Psychiatry, 17,* 203-213.

Stokes, T.F., and Baer, D.M. (1977). An implicit technology for generalization. *Journal of Applied Behavior Analysis, 10,* 349-367.

Sulzer-Azaroff, B., and Mayer, G.R. (1977). *Applying behavior-analysis procedures with children and youth.* New York: Holt, Rinehart and Winston.

Varni, J.W. (1983). *Clinical behavioral pediatrics: An interdisciplinary biobehavioral approach*. New York: Pergamon Press.

Watson, L.S. (1967). Application of operant conditioning techniques to institutionalized severely and profoundly retarded children. *Mental Retardation Abstracts, 4,* 1–18.

White, G.D., Nielson, G., and Johnson, S.M. (1972). Timeout duration and the suppression of deviant behavior in children. *Journal of Applied Behavior Analysis, 5,* 111–120.

CHAPTER 6

IDENTIFICATION AND EDUCATION OF CHILDREN AND ADOLESCENTS WITH LEARNING DISABILITIES, MENTAL RETARDATION, AND ORTHOPEDIC IMPAIRMENTS

Lois Therres Pommer

Since 1975, when Congress passed Public Law 94–142, the Education for All Handicapped Children Act, there has been a burgeoning interest in handicapped children, and a variety of diagnostic and educational programming techniques have been proposed for their identification and treatment. Now all professionals who work with children must be able to decide when to make a referral to determine if a child has a handicapping condition so that appropriate educational placement and instruction can occur. Furthermore, as the PL 94–142 concept of "least restrictive environment" for educating handicapped children is implemented, regular and special educators must be prepared to meet the educational needs of handicapped students.

A total of 4,363,031 handicapped students received federally mandated special education services during the 1984–85 school year (U.S. Department of Education, 1985). The most prevalent handicapping condition was learning disabilities, for which 1,839,292 students were served in the 1984–85 school year, an increase of 131 percent since 1976–77. This increase in children identified as learning disabled was accompanied by a 26 percent decrease in children reported as mentally retarded. In 1976–77, a total of 969,547 children were reported as mentally retarded; in 1984–85, a total of 717,785 mentally retarded children were reported. Orthopedically impaired children totalled 87,008 in 1976–77 and 58,835 in 1984–85, a decrease of 32 percent, which is partially explained by many orthopedically impaired children being reclassified as multihandicapped.

The type and extent of educational services available to these handicapped children vary according to the individual needs of each student and the array of services available in the school district. Most handicapped students receive the majority of their educational program in regular classes, although the extent to which this is true varies according to handicap. During the 1983–84 school year, 77 percent of learning disabled children were placed in regular education classes that were supplemented by special education services received outside the regular education class. This left 23 percent of learning disabled students in self-contained special education classes or separate schools. Mentally retarded children traditionally have been served in more restrictive settings. During the 1983–84 school year, only 30 percent of mentally retarded students were placed primarily in regular education, with another 54 percent being placed in self-contained special education classes held in a regular school, and 16 percent being placed in segregated special education schools or other specialized environments. During the same time period, 37 percent of orthopedically impaired students received most of their services in regular education, with an additional 38 percent being educated in self-contained special education classes in regular schools and 25 percent in segregated special education schools or other specialized environments.

LEARNING DISABILITIES

Gilly is an 8-year-old boy who attends the third grade in a local public school. Gilly's parents and teacher have expressed concern over his high activity level, inability to sit still, and easy distractibility. His academic skills are poor, particularly in reading, and his parents believe that he is "bright but lazy." They note that he avoids doing homework and does not like school. Gilly's peer relationships are unsatisfactory, with fights occurring almost daily. In their effort to understand and help Gilly, his teachers referred him for cognitive and academic testing.

Psychological testing with the Wechsler Intelligence Scale for Children–Revised (Wechsler, 1974) revealed overall intellectual functioning to be normal (Full Scale IQ, 97) but with a significant range of variability across areas. His performance on visual perception, visual memory, and visual-motor tasks fell in the mildly retarded range. In contrast, his short-term auditory memory was low average. When tasks required the use of both auditory and visual channels together, Gilly's performance was average. Strengths were exhibited in concrete and abstract reasoning skills. Academic testing, using the Woodcock-Johnson Psycho-Educational Test Battery (Woodcock and Johnson, 1977), revealed overall reading skills at the first grade level. An analysis of his reading performance showed that Gilly identified most letters, with a few reversals (p,q; b,d), read a few one-syllable words, and filled in a word in one sentence that was accompanied by a picture clue. No word analysis skills were exhibited. An Informal Reading Inventory was administered, and Gilly read a preprimer passage with comprehension but was frustrated at the primer level. When the examiner read stories aloud, Gilly demonstrated comprehension at the third grade level. His performance on the Mathematics Cluster of the Woodcock-Johnson test fell within low normal limits for his age, although he had specific difficulties in telling time. A writing sample was elicited, and Gilly wrote one brief sentence with errors, omitting punctuation and capitalization ("i was a bog in the stret" for "I saw a dog in the street"). He used manuscript letter formations of poor quality and varying sizes. During academic testing, Gilly was quite fidgety and required tangible reinforcers to complete his work.

An interdisciplinary team, consisting of Gilly's parents, developmental pediatrician, school psychologist, behavioral psychologist, educational evaluator, social worker, and Gilly's teacher, met to discuss school placement and programming. The team agreed that Gilly had a learning disability and required placement in a small, structured, self-contained class. Furthermore, because of Gilly's improved functioning when using auditory and visual channels in combination, they suggested that multisensory techniques be employed to aid Gilly in learning. The behavioral psychologist and classroom teacher agreed to develop a behavior management system to increase on-task behaviors and decrease behavioral outbursts. The team would meet 60 days after placement to review the effectiveness of the program. If Gilly continued to exhibit overactive, inattentive behaviors, the pediatrician would consider a trial of stimulant medication to be monitored by the parent and teacher.

Gilly is just one example of a learning disabled child. Children with learning disabilities are a diverse group, and the guidelines that define these children are quite broad.

Definition of Learning Disabilities

PL 94-142 provides the following definition of learning disabilities:

Specific learning disability means a disorder in one or more of the basic psychological processes involved in understanding or in using language, spoken or written, which may manifest itself in an imperfect ability to listen, think, speak, read, write, spell, or do mathematical calculations.

The term [specific learning disability] includes such conditions as perceptual handicaps, brain injury, minimal brain dysfunction, dyslexia, and developmental aphasia. The term does not include children who have learning problems which are primarily the result of visual, hearing, or motor handicaps, of mental retardation, or of environmental, cultural, or economic disadvantage.

Although "severe discrepancy" does not appear in the PL 94-142 definition of learning disability, most states have used some criteria to define a severe discrepancy between ability and achievement to limit the number of children identified as learning disabled. These criteria are often shaped by budgetary constraints rather than by ideological convictions. To limit the children served under PL 94-142, guidelines for "severe discrepancy" were published in the *Federal Register* in 1977 (U.S. Office of Education, 1977). Severe discrepancy between achievement and intellectual ability must be documented in one or more of these areas: (1) oral expression; (2) listening comprehension; (3) written expression; (4) basic reading skill; (5) reading comprehension; (6) mathematics calculation; or (7) mathematics reasoning (U.S. Office of Education, 1977). Although the extent of the ability-achievement discrepancy required to define a child as learning disabled varies from state to state, the criterion of "2 years below grade level" has been used frequently (Chalfant, 1984; Shepard, 1983). The difficulty in using this criterion is that 2 years below grade level is quite different for a third grade student than for a twelfth grade student in terms of severity and impact. In fact, a 1 year discrepancy at third grade level is probably a greater handicap than a 2 year discrepancy at twelfth grade level. Moreover, the child's intellectual ability may not be taken into account, thus commingling slow learners and learning disabled children.

Despite the variations among learning disabled students, some commonalities can be isolated. A student who is diagnosed as learning disabled must fulfill the following criteria in most states:

1. Intelligence falls within the average range.
2. A discrepancy exists between intelligence and academic achievement.
3. The discrepancy between intelligence and academic achievement is not caused by other primary factors (i.e., visual, hearing, or motor handicaps, mental retardation, emotional disturbance, or environmental, cultural, or economic disadvantage).
4. A dysfunction exists in learning processes.

Although there is much professional debate as to how to define learning disabilities, at this time a combination of the PL 94-142 definition and the federal guidelines on severe discrepancy is commonly used. Whether or not an individual student meets these criteria for having a learning disability is determined through evaluation of the student.

Evaluation of Learning Disabled Students

Clinicians have experienced difficulty in differentiating some learning disabled students from those who are emotionally disturbed, especially among adolescents. Learning disabled children who are not identified or provided with appropriate instructional programming become frustrated and develop a poor self-concept, which often leads to either aggression or withdrawal.

Learning disabled students who exhibit aggressive behaviors are more likely to be referred for an assessment and, therefore, are more likely to be diagnosed as learning disabled. Those who withdraw are less likely to be noticed by the teacher and referred for testing. In any case, the clinician is left to ponder whether the learning disabled child became emotionally disturbed because of difficulty in learning or whether the child failed to learn because of his or her emotional disturbance.

Formal and Informal Assessment

The most critical factor in educational planning is a good diagnostic study, which employs formal and informal techniques to determine intelligence, academic levels, memory skills, attentional skills, social skills, motor functioning, adaptive behavior, language, and emotional status. All of this information is combined to reach a diagnosis, which is then used to determine an appropriate school placement and to tailor learning experiences to the specific needs of the student.

It is important to use appropriate standardized tests to measure the intelligence and achievement of handicapped children to avoid bias and inappropriate placement and to enhance programming. At a minimum, an assessment for learning disabilities will include the following: (1) intelligence testing, (2) academic testing, and (3) other assessments as deemed necessary (medical, physical, speech, language, emotional, behavioral, ophthalmological, audiological, and neurological).

For a child to be considered learning disabled, there must be a severe discrepancy between the results of intelligence testing and academic testing in oral expression, listening comprehension, written expression, basic reading skills, reading comprehension, mathematics calculation, or mathematics reasoning.

In addition to using standardized tests to assess learning disabilities and suggest appropriate instructional programming, qualitative data should also be examined and considered. Classroom observations should be used to generate a systematic accounting of on-task behaviors, off-task behaviors, activity level, concentration, organizational skills, impulse control, and attending behaviors, as well as academic performance.

Furthermore, it is particularly important to consider pedagogy and look at what teaching techniques have been used in the past to determine what has been successful and what has failed. Samples of class work, information on the family, cultural and environmental background, developmental history, and reports from teachers are crucial in diagnosing and planning an approach for a learning disabled student.

Components of Written Reports

Written reports used to establish the presence of a learning disability should contain the following components:

1. A diagnosis of learning disability.
2. A statement of the criteria used to determine the existence of a learning disability.
3. A description of deviations from developmental milestones and general educational objectives.
4. An indication that the severe discrepancy between intelligence and achievement requires special educational services.
5. A description of the perceptual and cognitive functioning indicative of a learning disability.
6. A description of relevant behaviors from observations of the student.
7. An indication of the relationship of the student's behavior to his or her academic functioning.
8. Educationally relevant medical information (when applicable).
9. A determination of the effects of environmental, cultural, or economic disadvantage.

Teaching Approaches for Learning Disabled Students

Because learning disabled students are a heterogeneous group, there is no *one* instructional method or curriculum that is appropriate for all. In fact, a key characteristic of learning disabled students is that they do not learn from standard instruction in one or more academic areas. Students may spend years "failing" in school and developing emotional problems—often avoiding academic work by overt defiance, clowning, sitting in silence, or "looking busy." While many learning disabled students have been denounced as lazy or as showing little effort, learning disabled students are not inherently lazy. With standard instruction, however, they would not be able to learn at their potential no matter how hard they tried. When instruction is given in a way in which the learning disabled student can be successful, his or her effort increases significantly.

After a diagnosis of learning disability has been made, the teachers, with the help of other professionals and the parents, must determine how to instruct the student. Most learning disabled students benefit from multisensory instruction, but some students are basically visual learners, and some are basically auditory learners; as a consequence, the actual teaching methods that may be used with learning disabled students are limitless. An individualized educational program must be developed to allow each student to learn at his or her own speed. For each learning disabled child, the teacher must look for appropriate instructional content, methods, and materials to educate and provide remediation in specific disability areas. Small pupil-teacher ratios are essential because of the distractibility and short attention span seen in many of these children, as well as the need for individual instruction and monitoring of learning disabled students. The following are broad instructional suggestions for teachers who work with learning disabled children.

- Provide focus and informative feedback.
- Provide repetition and practice.
- Provide training for transfer.
- Provide consistency in directions.
- Provide consistency in behavioral management.
- Reward positive behavior.
- Use motivational materials.
- Provide multiple approaches for instruction.
- Make environmental adaptations.
- Reduce environmental distractions.
- Accommodate individual differences in intellectual potential, sensory ability, modality strengths and weaknesses, attentional skills, and need for reinforcement and support.

The teacher must act as an effective instructional manager to elicit acceptable behavior from students. The likelihood of obtaining appropriate classroom behavior is enhanced by having a standard class routine and developing a set way of dealing with inappropriate behaviors and resolving conflicts. Moreover, the teacher needs to select appropriate content and methods of instruction. The content should be as interesting and personally meaningful as possible for the students, and the methods of presentation should be varied, utilizing the sensory and processing strengths of the students. The teacher should communicate goals to the students, and progression toward those goals should be monitored carefully. Furthermore, the teacher needs to help the students *see* the progress they are making. Finally, each student's readiness to advance to a higher level of instruction must be evaluated carefully.

Computer technology presents many advantages in the educational instruction of learning disabled students. These benefits include immediate feedback and reinforcement, development of skills in attending, development of skills in following directions, hierarchical instruction, with subprograms if a lesson is not mastered, and little requirement for social interaction. Pommer, Mark, and Hayden (1983) have provided an overview on how to view computer software as an effective adjunct to the curricula for learning disabled students. More special education software needs to be developed, particularly in the area of logical thinking and memory, but the possibilities for the use of computers with learning disabled students are limitless.

Although it is apparent that not all learning disabled children benefit from the same teaching approach, implementation of these general recommendations in tandem with individualized instructional strategies and appropriate content will promote student learning.

Medical Treatment of Attentional Deficits in Learning Disabled Students

A major issue in the field of learning disabilities is the use of stimulant drug treatment to alleviate symptoms of attention deficit disorders. Recent figures estimate that 1 to 2 percent of America's school-age population is currently being treated with stimulant medication (Breger, 1981). This involves as many as 600,000 or more children, a 400 percent increase over 1970 (Kavale, 1982). Attention-deficit hyperactivity disorder and its treatment are discussed more fully in Chapters 2, 3, and 4.

The most common method of determining if medication is needed for children with ADHD and of subsequently assessing the effectiveness of drug therapy is the use of rating scales completed by teachers or parents, or both. Thus, the outcome of drug therapy ultimately is judged by teachers and parents. One of the best scales for evaluating the effects of drug therapy is Conners' Teacher Rating Scale (Conners, 1969), which provides information on the child's activity level, attention span, concentration, and relevant personality variables. This scale is reproduced in Figure 2-1.

Review of the Research on Stimulant Drugs

Some children with attention-deficit hyperactivity disorder do not respond to drug therapy, but there are no clear-cut guidelines as to who will respond and who will not respond (Wender and Wender, 1978). Some factors postulated to influence drug response include the age of the child, the severity of the attentional deficits, evidence of organic involvement, parental style, and family psychopathology.

Barkley (1977) reviewed studies on children diagnosed as having attention deficit disorders. He studied 48 examples of research, and found that 75 percent of the children improved on stimulant medication, whereas for 25 percent the disorder remained unchanged or worsened. Some researchers demonstrated improvement on short-term memory tasks when the children were on drug treatment. They attributed improved short-term memory to improved attention and concentration (Sprague and Sleator, 1977). Another study (Flintoff, Barron, Swanson, Ledlow, and Kinsbourne, 1982) demonstrated greatly improved attention on a visual scanning task while the children were taking methylphenidate. Specifically, the children looked more frequently at the stimulus, made more comparisons, and selected a larger number of variants for comparison. Other studies have indicated that stimulants improve concentration as measured by continuous attention tasks (Conners and Rothchild, 1968; Sykes, Douglas, and Morgenstern, 1972). Denhoff, Davids, and Hawkins (1971) showed that dextroamphetamine sulfate improved the child's level of activity, length of attention span, and level of impulsivity. Studies by Gittelman-Klein and coworkers (1976) have demonstrated that drug treatment is more effective than behavioral management techniques in improving attention and concentration as defined by in-seat, on-task behaviors. Loney (1979) also found drug treatment to be more effective than other techniques in producing on-task behaviors.

Yet, despite all the research findings about children's improved attention and concentration, corresponding academic gains have not been shown. Gadow (1981) emphasized that there is no connection between improved attention and concentration and improved school learning, school performance, or solving of complex tasks. It may be that medication improves attention and behavior, but it does not compensate for the poor academic skills of the attention deficit disordered, learning disabled child.

A study by Firestone (1982) explored attitudes toward stimulant medication. Firestone located 76 children who met the criteria for attention deficit disorder and whom he believed would benefit from drug therapy. Twenty-six percent of the families refused drug treatment for their children. By the end of 4 months, 20 percent of those agreeing to drug therapy had discontinued its use. By the end of 10 months, only 55 percent of the original group remained on stimulant drugs. Firestone also noted that only 10 percent of the families contacted the physician prior to discontinuing medication. Firestone concluded that the parents and teachers of many children with attention deficit disorder do not accept treatment with stimulant medication.

Sleator, Ullmann, and von Neumann (1982) interviewed 52 children with attention deficit disorder who were receiving drug therapy and had been on drug treatment for at least 1 year. They found that 31 percent of the children believed that the drug helped only a little bit, and an additional 27 percent thought that the drug did not help at all in terms of concentration, getting work done, and paying attention. They also noted that 42 percent of the children hated or disliked taking stimulant medication, 29 percent were indifferent to it, and only 29 percent had positive feelings.

Children have devised a variety of ways to avoid taking stimulant medication, including arguing with parents, outright refusal, throwing the medication away when others were not looking, deliberately forgetting to remind parents or teachers, and ''cheeking'' their medication and disposing of it later. It is imperative that cooperation be elicited from any child being given a stimulant drug and that the attitudes of parents and teachers be considered. Without the combined cooperation of parents, teachers, and children, stimulant medication will be less than fully effective.

MENTAL RETARDATION

Roni was a premature baby, born at 36 weeks' gestation and weighing 4 pounds, 3 ounces. There was a low level of fetal activity throughout the pregnancy. Just after birth, Roni developed severe anemia and required a blood transfusion. She was discharged from the hospital in good condition at 4 weeks, when she reached the weight of 5 pounds. Roni's infancy was remarkable for excessive sleeping and poor feeding. Developmental milestones indicated some delays and deviance. In the gross motor area, she rolled over prone to supine at 5 months, sat unsupported at 9 months, cruised at 14 months, and walked unassisted at 21 months. Currently, at the age of 5 years, Roni is unable to ride a tricycle. In fine motor skills, she demonstrated a voluntary grasp at 5 to 6 months and finger-thumb apposition at 11 months. She could spoon feed with some spilling at 24 months. Currently, she can dress herself except for zippers, buttons, and shoelaces. She was bladder trained at 3 to 4 years but was not bowel trained until this year (age 5 years). In language, she had a social smile at 3 months, oriented to voice at 4 months, was cooing at 6 months, used gestures to communicate at 14 months, said "mama" and "dada" specifically at 2 years, used a few single words at 3 years, and combined words at 4 years. Roni now speaks in phrases and brief sentences of 3 to 4 words.

She entered a regular kindergarten at 5 years of age. Her teacher noted that Roni was passive and lacked such skills as color and shape recognition. In school, the teacher found that Roni's progress was far slower than that of other students. After 2 months of school, the teacher referred Roni to the school psychologist for testing. Results on the Wechsler Preschool and Primary Scales of Intelligence (Wechsler, 1967) revealed a Full Scale IQ of 60, with a Verbal IQ of 58 and a Performance IQ of 61, thus placing her in the mildly retarded range. Results of the Vineland Adaptive Behavior Scales (Sparrow, Balla, and Cicchetti, 1984) indicated delays in the acquisition of adaptive skills. Educational testing, using the Developmental Activities Screening Inventory (Fewell and Langley, 1984), Learning Accomplishment Profile (Lemay, Griffin, and Sanford, 1977), and selected subtests from the Brigance Diagnostic Inventory of Early Development (Brigance, 1977), showed that Roni's preacademic skills were commensurate with her intellectual level. The school interdisciplinary team met and determined that Roni should receive special education programming, with an emphasis on adaptive-functional behaviors and use of a developmental approach.

Roni is an example of a mildly mentally retarded child. There is a range of mental retardation, and much individual variation exists within that range. Throughout the following section, the diversity in levels of mental retardation will be explored.

Definition of Mental Retardation

According to Public Law 94-142, mental retardation is defined as follows:

> Mentally retarded means significantly sub-average general intellectual functioning, existing concurrently with deficits in adaptive behavior and manifested during the developmental period, which adversely affects a child's educational performance.

In this definition of mental retardation, "significantly sub-average intellectual functioning" means a score that falls two standard deviations below the mean on a major standardized test of intelligence. The Wechsler Preschool and Primary Scale of Intelligence (Wechsler, 1967), Wechsler Intelligence Scale for Children—Revised (Wechsler, 1974), and

Kaufman Assessment Battery for Children (Kaufman and Kaufman, 1983), three frequently used and individually administered tests of intelligence, have a mean of 100 and a standard deviation of 15. Another commonly used intelligence measure, the Stanford-Binet Intelligence Scale (Thorndike, Hagen, and Sattler, 1986), has a mean of 100 and a standard deviation of 16. Mildly retarded persons have an IQ falling in the range of 50–55 to approximately 69; moderately retarded persons have an IQ in the 35–40 to 50–55 range; severely retarded persons have an IQ falling in the 20–25 to 35–40 range; and profoundly retarded persons have an IQ falling below 20–25. Approximately 2 to 3 percent of the population have IQ scores below 70. This scoring system uses the same IQ number divisions as the American Association on Mental Deficiency (AAMD) classification (American Association on Mental Deficiency, 1983).

The term "developmental period" from the PL 94-142 definition of mental retardation is considered to be the first 18 years. "Adaptive behavior" is the degree to which the person can function independently and be socially responsible in his or her environment. Instruments such as the Vineland Adaptive Behavior Scales (Sparrow, Balla, and Cicchetti, 1984), Woodcock-Johnson Scales of Independent Behavior (Bruininks, Woodcock, Weatherman, and Hill, 1984), and AAMD Adaptive Behavior Scale (Nihira, Foster, Shellhaas, and Leland, 1975) are commonly used, standardized measures of adaptive functioning. Specific areas surveyed include social interaction, eating, toileting, money skills, time skills, self-help skills, and communication skills. Both cognitive level and adaptive level must be considered in deciding whether or not a child is retarded. Levels of adaptive functioning are particularly important in light of possible social-cultural discrimination of intelligence tests.

Levels of retardation generally are discussed according to severity and expectations for the person's academic and overall development. The majority of retarded persons have mild degrees of retardation and will achieve academic skills at the third to sixth grade level. Nearly all mildly retarded persons can live independently as adults and support themselves. Moderately retarded persons (0.3 percent of the total population) will achieve academic skills at the kindergarten to third grade level, and they can learn to care for themselves and live in the community with some supervision and assistance. Severely and profoundly retarded persons constitute only 0.1 percent of the total population. Most severely retarded persons function between the 2- and five-year-old level. They can learn to care for some of their own needs and can be employed in a sheltered workshop. Profoundly retarded persons generally function between the level of birth and 2 years and will need a great deal of supervision; however, often they can learn some self-care skills (e.g., feeding and dressing). The extent to which retarded persons function independently is a consequence not only of level of retardation but also of their education.

Evaluation of Mentally Retarded Students

The medical doctor's skills in observing the preschool child's development will often determine whether or not a young mentally retarded child is identified as such. The physician has access to the child's developmental history and has examined the child physically, neurologically, and developmentally. The physician may notice deviations or delays in the child's development, and, at times, the physical examination may reveal a specific syndrome associated with mental retardation. For some children the physician may ascertain that there is developmental and neurological deterioration. In any of these cases, the physician should refer the child for comprehensive developmental testing.

Formal and Informal Assessment

To plan and implement an effective instructional program, formal and informal assessments are needed. Information regarding intelligence, receptive and expressive language, academic levels, motor functioning, social skills, and adaptive behavior must be considered in individualizing the school program according to the needs of the student.

Two assessments are essential to make a diagnosis of mental retardation: intelligence testing and adaptive behavior measure. When considered together, intelligence and adaptive behavior assessments determine whether or not a child is retarded and then classify the child according to the degree of retardation. One purpose of intelligence testing is to provide a measurement of the child's general intellectual level. A second purpose is to obtain a profile of individual strengths and weaknesses, which can be used to develop an instructional plan. The measure of adaptive behavior is used to help determine the level of retardation and to determine the extent to which the student is independent and socially sufficient in his or her own environment. Knowledge of adaptive skills is essential for curriculum development.

In addition to testing intelligence and adaptive functioning, educational achievement testing is desirable for mentally retarded youngsters and helps the classroom teacher select and implement appropriate classroom activities. The need for additional assessments (i.e., medical, physical, vocational, speech, language, emotional, behavioral, ophthalmological, audiological, and neurological) must be decided on a case-by-case basis.

Besides the results of formal testing, information gathered from informal assessments is beneficial in assessing the educational needs of mentally retarded students. Informal assessments include classroom observations, developmental history, reports from teachers, samples of class work, past pedagogy, and information on family, cultural, and environmental background. An analysis of the student's current living situation and current self-help or functional skills will help determine the content that should be taught in the classroom and used in school, home, and community to help the child or adolescent function as independently as possible.

Components of Written Reports

Written reports establishing that the child is mentally retarded should contain the following components:

1. A diagnosis of mental retardation
2. A statement of the criteria used to determine retardation
3. A classification of level of retardation (mild, moderate, severe, or profound)
4. A description of adaptive functioning indicative of mental retardation
5. Relevant behaviors from observations of the student
6. Educationally relevant medical information
7. Educationally relevant information from other sources (e.g., speech, language, vocational, behavioral, emotional)

When considered together, all of these findings provide the basis for determining appropriate teaching strategies.

Teaching Approaches for Mentally Retarded Students

To plan an instructional program for a mentally retarded student, information in these areas is crucial: assessment results, adaptive behavior, adaptive requirements in the student's environment, level of cognition, and interests of the student.

Any curriculum for a mentally retarded child should include leisure education, which means educating the child on "wholesome use of discretionary time in order to enhance the quality of one's life" (Bender, Brannan, and Verhoven, 1984). It also should include self-help, safety, and social skills. Even in elementary school years, teachers must consider eventual work placement and ways to facilitate personal independence.

In designing a functional-prevocational curriculum, the teacher must "conceptualize those general behaviors that are critical to successful independent functioning" (Bender and Valletutti, 1985). The teacher must then identify specific skills to be taught, keeping in mind their functional utility. Bender and Valletutti provide a specific curriculum framework for teaching functional activities. A skill sequence must be established through a task analysis of what is to be learned. Thus, the teacher breaks down each task into small steps, each step building on the preceding one. It is imperative that the teacher use concrete objects, chronologically age-appropriate materials and activities and natural settings. For example, in teaching retarded students how to identify the word "toilet," the teacher should have students locate the word in a specific bathroom in the school. They should then identify a toilet in a different bathroom in the school and finally in a bathroom in the community. As generalization does not occur automatically for retarded students, the teacher must plan for it. In the example above, if the word "toilet" were only taught in relation to one bathroom, the mentally retarded student might not recognize it in other settings. Therefore, the teacher must use multiple examples and multiple settings in order to promote generalization.

Another principle in designing an instructional program for retarded students is the concept of partial participation. In this situation, materials and procedures are adapted to enable students to take some part in activities they cannot perform independently. For example, if a retarded student cannot learn to heat a can of soup, perhaps he or she can learn to select a can of soup from the cupboard and hand it to another person for preparation.

In providing an appropriate instructional program for retarded students, the teacher must also understand and use such behavior modification principles as reinforcement and extinction, as well as techniques of shaping, modeling, fading, and time out. The teacher must keep in mind that behavior is learned on the basis of its consequences and that behavior that produces gratifying results will recur.

Inappropriate behaviors exhibited by some severely or profoundly retarded persons may include sterotyped movements such as rocking, intricate hand movements, gazing at objects such as lights, hair twirling, or thumb sucking. To decrease socially inappropriate behaviors and increase appropriate behaviors, the teacher must design a behavior management plan and review its effectiveness. Measurements must be taken of the child's behavior before beginning an intervention program, during treatment, and after treatment. If the frequency and duration of inappropriate behavior decreases, the teacher should continue with the program. If the frequency and duration of inappropriate behavior remains the same or increases, a new behavior management plan must be developed. A more detailed discussion of the use of behavioral interventions with handicapped youngsters is presented in Chapter 5.

Many mentally retarded persons present an image of helplessness. This may result from years of experience of being retarded and from being in overly protective settings (Rosen, Clark, and Kivitz, 1977).

Thus, many retarded persons become too acquiescent and compliant, which makes them easy targets for exploitation. Furthermore, retarded people may demonstrate poor ability to adapt to new situations. Two critically important principles are needed to increase flexibility and feelings of competence and control for the retarded person: (1) normalization of experiences, and (2) acquisition of adaptive or functional behaviors. Simply stated, normalization is letting mentally retarded persons obtain an experience as close to the normal as possible (Nirje, 1969). Normalization occurs only with the acquisition of adaptive or functional behaviors, which equip the retarded person for maximum independence. These adaptive or functional behaviors include skills in self-care, communication, fine motor, gross motor, and housekeeping.

The use of computers with the mentally retarded offers hope for improving quality of life and achieving increased independence. A major benefit of using computer technology is the opportunity it gives the mentally retarded to exert some control over their environment. Project ACTT (Activating Children Through Technology) has developed ways to connect switch-activated toys to the computer to promote knowledge of cause-effect relationships. The Association for Retarded Citizens is developing a device that will indicate when the bladder is full. Initially, the teacher or other adult will take responsibility for tracking the bladder-sensing signal and taking the retarded person to the bathroom. The retarded person will then be taught to recognize the signal. Next, he or she will be taught both to recognize the signal and go to the bathroom. Finally, the retarded person will learn to recognize the physical signs that the bladder is full. More steps can be added to this process, if needed. Some retarded persons will never reach the goal of independent toileting, but they will reach their functioning potential.

When mentally retarded persons are taught functional skills, their natural daily performance and contact with these skills will help to maintain them. Furthermore, the acquisition of functional skills permits the retarded person to have more control over his or her environment, which in turn increases his or her dignity and acceptance by others.

Seizures

Seizure disorders may be associated with mental retardation, although most retarded people do not have them. For those retarded students who have seizures, the teacher, physician, and parents must work together to manage the seizures with the goal of achieving maximum seizure control and minimum side effects. The student with a seizure disorder may require support and assistance in adjusting to the seizures. The teacher should analyze instructional tasks to ensure safety and consult with a medical doctor if there are any questions as to whether or not particular tasks are dangerous to the person with seizures or to classmates and teachers. For example, it may be dangerous to allow a person with a seizure disorder to operate certain machinery in industrial arts class.

ORTHOPEDIC IMPAIRMENTS

Michael was born after a 40-week uncomplicated pregnancy. Fetal activity was noted at 4 months. Labor began spontaneously, and the infant required delivery by forceps. After delivery, Michael was limp and cyanotic (blue in color), without spontaneous respirations. Suctioning and positive pressure bagging were used to resuscitate him. By 10 minutes after birth, his respiratory rate was within normal limits. Further neonatal complications included the development of abnormal posturing and seizure activity at 42 hours of age.

During infancy, Michael's sucking reflex was poor. At the age of 12 months, his parents took him to a developmental clinic because of his inability to sit or crawl. This initial evaluation revealed significantly delayed gross motor skills with better upper extremity control on the left than on the right. He was diagnosed as having cerebral palsy. His subsequent developmental history included sitting with support at $2\frac{1}{2}$ years, cruising with assistance at $4\frac{1}{2}$ years, and crawling at 7 years. In the fine motor area, Michael first reached out for objects at 6 months, grasped objects at 2 years, finger fed at $2\frac{1}{2}$ years, and cooperated with dressing at $3\frac{1}{2}$ years. Language milestones were within normal limits.

Michael began attending a special education school for orthopedically impaired children at 2 years of age. At the age of 5 years, the school psychologist determined that Michael had normal intelligence. Testing was also conducted by an occupational therapist, a physical therapist, and an educational evaluator. An interdisciplinary team determined that Michael should be enrolled in a regular kindergarten with resource services from occupational therapy and physical therapy.

Currently, Michael is 10 years old and in a regular fifth grade class with occupational and physical therapy as resource services. He can transfer without help from his wheelchair to his classroom chair, and he transfers from his wheelchair to the ground with minimal assistance. On floor mats Michael is learning to "knee walk," bearing weight on his upper extremities. His stability is poor, and he tends to fall backward. He requires some assistance with dressing and undressing. The broad goals of occupational therapy and physical therapy are to maximize his functional capacity to live independently.

In their concern for Michael, who is an only child, his parents have tended to protect him and provide assistance in tasks he could perform independently. Recently, the school social worker, occupational therapist, and physical therapist met with the parents to discuss Michael's need to separate, both physically and emotionally, from his parents. His parents expressed their need for guidance and support, and they agreed to obtain private family counseling through the local cerebral palsy organization. The team decided that Michael should also receive individual counseling to deal with his feelings of being "different" and "helpless," feelings which were conditioned both by his handicap and by years of being overly protected. Moreover, the team recommended that Michael be integrated more fully into his community, including recreation programs.

Cerebral palsy is just one of many impairments that have an orthopedic component. The type of physical disability, the extent of disability, and the need for specialized services vary from child to child.

Definition of Orthopedic Impairment

PL 94-142 provides a definition of orthopedic impairment that is used for identification of need and provision of educational services.

> Orthopedically impaired means a severe orthopedic impairment which adversely affects a child's educational performance. The term includes impairments caused by congenital anomaly (for example, clubfoot, absence of some member, etc.), impairments caused by disease (for example, poliomyelitis, bone tuberculosis, etc.), and impairments from other causes (for example, cerebral palsy, amputations, and fractures or burns which cause contractures).

The key component in identifying a child as orthopedically impaired and requiring special educational services is that the orthopedic impairment adversely affects a child's *educational* performance. If there is no adverse effect on educational performance, a child with an orthopedic impairment would not qualify for a special education placement or ancillary services.

Evaluation of Orthopedically Impaired Students

As with learning disabilities and mental retardation, a combination of formal and informal techniques is needed. Assessment of orthopedically impaired children will determine intelligence, academic levels, type and extent of orthopedic handicap, adaptive behavior, and degree to which the impairment affects the child's educational program.

In developing a test battery for an orthopedically impaired child, many evaluators use a "cafeteria" approach, taking selected items from various tests, depending upon the child's handicaps. Bender and Pommer (1984) have suggested specific tests and possible modifications that are useful with this population. In assessing the intelligence and academic skill levels of an orthopedically impaired child, the evaluator must differentiate between the child's cognition and skills and his or her physical ability to demonstrate that knowledge to the evaluator. For some orthopedically impaired children, the test may reflect their disability more than their ability. As noted by Anastasi (1982), "Informal adjustments in testing procedures [must be] made in order to adapt the test to the child's response capacities." Although any adaptations made in the standardized instructions for a test reduce the validity of the test results, it is not productive to require more than the child's physical capabilities allow. For example, if a child has a motor impairment that prevents him or her from pointing to the correct response, the evaluator may elect to use eye gaze as a response. For some orthopedically impaired children, the evaluator may manipulate test materials such as puzzles according to the student's verbal instructions or head movements. Another common modification is an extension of time limits. Although these modifications are essential, there is little research regarding the methodological effects of deviating from standardized test instructions. Decisions about deviations must then rely on the clinical judgment of the evaluator.

Referrals for occupational therapy are often made because of difficulty in the fine motor area; obvious perceptual or perceptual-motor problems; general clumsiness; positioning problems and the need for adaptive equipment; difficulty with chewing or swallowing; and inability to effectively eat independently (Exner, 1986). Some common reasons for referrals for physical therapy include poor or absent sitting posture or head control, asymmetry, atrophy, musculoskeletal or neuromuscular disability, delayed developmental milestone achievement, poor motor control, disturbed balance, perceptual dysfunction, absence of a limb or traumatic amputation, scoliosis, and confinement to a wheelchair (Esterson, 1986). Evaluations performed by medical doctors, occupational therapists, and physical therapists should provide a diagnostic label, a description of the child's physical capabilities and limitations, an indication of how the orthopedic impairment affects educational performance, and educational programming recommendations.

Qualitative assessment data to be considered along with quantitative test data include the child's emotional or behavioral reactions to his or her orthopedic impairment, peer relationships, developmental history, past pedagogy, reports from teachers, classroom behavior, class work, and information on the child's family, cultural, and environmental background. Some indication of the child's dependency level, self-esteem, and frustration tolerance is imperative. All of this information, together with reports of cognitive and academic testing and reports of medical or physical handicaps, is essential in formulating an appropriate educational program and planning effective instruction.

Medical doctors are in the best position to locate and refer children with orthopedic impairments, although teachers, parents, school nurses, and others may do so. Any necessary medication is prescribed by the physician; however, therapists, teachers, parents, and others may be asked to monitor the effects of medication. Relevant data regarding the child's physical abilities, disabilities, and limitations should be conveyed to the classroom teacher by the physical therapist, occupational therapist, or physician. Any medical or other technical terms used to describe or treat the orthopedically impaired child must be translated into layman's terms for all who are involved in the child's education.

Components of Written Reports

Written reports used to establish the special education needs of orthopedically impaired students should contain the following components:

1. An indication of the specific orthopedic impairment.
2. Statements regarding the impact of the orthopedic impairment on educational performance.
3. A description of physical capabilities and limitations that affect educational programming.
4. Statements regarding any other factors that affect educational performance (e.g., cognition, behavioral difficulties, emotional status).
5. Need for any environmental adaptations (e.g., modifications needed for wheelchair access).
6. Need for any adaptive materials or devices (e.g., specialized head gear, splints, prone boards).

To make appropriate school placement decisions for orthopedically impaired children, the interdisciplinary team must have all of the foregoing information in writing from qualified professionals. Moreover, teachers need this information to plan classroom activities and select suitable teaching strategies.

Teaching Approaches for Orthopedically Impaired Students

The cardinal rule in planning the educational program of orthopedically impaired students is to treat them as much like their nonhandicapped peers as possible. Some modifications may be necessary, however. Classrooms must be accessible to the wheelchair-bound student. Therapists or other qualified personnel need to show the classroom teacher how to transfer a wheelchair-bound student into a chair, if appropriate, and how to assist the student in the bathroom. Therapeutic positioning of the child may also be necessary in the classroom. Other physical and occupational therapy activities may include working on balance, range of motion, transfer skills, oral motor skills, fine motor skills (e.g., writing or cutting with scissors), and gross motor skills (e.g., ambulation). These activities may occur in individual or group sessions with a therapist, in sessions with a teacher or therapy assistant, or in the classroom with the teacher receiving consultative services from the therapist. Ongoing consultation and collaboration between the therapists and teachers is crucial if maximum progress is to be made.

Special note should be made of the importance of collaboration on activities of daily living (ADL), which are the skills that the child needs to have to function as normally as possible in his or her environment. ADL skills include eating, dressing, toileting, and personal hygiene. Therapists, teachers, parents, and, when appropriate, the child himself or herself should work together in developing, implementing, and monitoring the total educational program.

Facilitating Independence

As with mentally retarded persons, orthopedically impaired children often are overprotected by others in their environment. This overprotection generates dependency and thwarts the child's ability to function at maximum independence. All those who come into contact with orthopedically impaired students must be educated about the importance of promoting and facilitating independence. For example, if a child is learning to use a wheelchair and runs into walls, that child must be allowed to move the wheelchair away from the wall if he or she is capable of doing so. Others should not "rescue" the child by moving the wheelchair to the center of the corridor or wheeling the child to his or her destination. The acquisition of increased independence greatly improves the quality of life of the orthopedically impaired child.

Teachers, therapists, parents, and others should investigate leisure time activities and interests of orthopedically impaired children and promote appropriate, diversified, effective use of personal time. Bender, Brannan and Verhoven (1984) have developed an excellent curriculum guide in the area of leisure education.

Counseling is sometimes needed to deal with issues of self-concept. The orthopedically impaired person may need assistance in accepting himself or herself as a complete, valuable person with some physical limitations. As the student acquires more adaptive living skills and satisfying leisure time activities and thus becomes more independent, his or her self-esteem may increase.

Technology

Current and future possibilities for the use of technology with orthopedically impaired persons are wide and promising. For example, for persons who do not have the physical capability to feed themselves, a self-feeding tray is being explored. This tray would have three sections for different foods. The handicapped person would need only to move his or her head forward toward the food he or she wanted, and the device would fill a spoon with that food and bring it to mouth level, thus giving the person control over food selection and rate of speed at which he or she wants to eat.

Computers can increase independence for orthopedically impaired children and allow more choices and better control. Further information regarding the many types of computers available for the disabled can be found in *Communication, Control, and Computer Access for Disabled and Elderly Individuals* (Brandenberg and Vanderheiden, 1987).

SUMMARY

There are various ways to identify and program for the educational needs of learning disabled, mentally retarded, and orthopedically impaired children. This chapter uses PL 94-142 definitions as a basis and describes the types of educational settings in which children with these problems are placed. Detailed illustrative case histories are provided for each of these handicaps and include educational placement and programming decisions made by interdisciplinary teams. This chapter provides lists of the essential components of evaluations, including process, content, and report writing. Suggested teaching approaches for each handicap are offered. Medical treatment, behavior management, and technological aspects are also discussed.

School systems strive to develop and use appropriate identification criteria and instructional methods for the children they serve. As pointed out throughout this chapter, the ways in which children with identical handicapping labels differ from one another makes these tasks more complex, but some commonalities do exist. With input from various professionals, as well as parents and students, the educational needs of learning disabled, mentally retarded, and orthopedically impaired students can be met.

REFERENCES

American Association on Mental Deficiency. (1983). *Classification in mental retardation*. Washington, DC: Author.

Anastasi, A.L. (1982). *Psychological testing (5th ed.)*. New York: Macmillan.

Barkley, R.A. (1977). A review of stimulant drug research with hyperactive children. *Journal of Child Psychology and Psychiatry, 18,* 137–155.

Bender, M., Brannan, S., and Verhoven, P. (1984). *Leisure education for the handicapped: Curriculum goals, activities, and resources*. San Diego, California: College-Hill Press.

Bender, M., and Pommer, L. (1984). Psychological tests and methods for handicapped children. *Jornadas Internacionales,* 115–129.

Bender, M., and Valletutti, P. (1985). *Teaching the moderately and severely handicapped: Curriculum objectives, strategies, and activities*. Austin, Texas: Pro-Ed.

Brandenberg, S.A. & Vanderheiden, G.C. (Eds.). (1987). *Communication, control, and computer access for disabled and elderly individuals*: ResourceBooks 1–3. San Diego, California: College-Hill Press.

Breger, E. (1981). Drug treatment of hyperactivity: An ethical controversy. *U.S. Navy Medicine, 72* (11), 18–20.

Brigance, A. (1977). *Brigance diagnostic inventory of basic skills*. Woburn, Massachusetts: Curriculum Associates.

Bruininks, R.H., Woodcock, R.W., Weatherman, R.F., and Hill, B.K. (1984). *Woodcock-Johnson psycho-educational battery, part 4: Scales of independent behavior*. Allen, Texas: Teaching Resources.

Chalfant, J. (1984). *Identifying learning disabled students: Guidelines for decision making*. Burlington, Vermont: Northeast Regional Resource Center (NERRC).

Conners, C.K. (1969). A teacher rating scale for use in drug studies with children. *American Journal of Psychiatry, 126,* 884–888.

Conners, C.K., and Rothschild, G.H. (1968). Drugs and learning in children. In J. Hellmuth (Ed.), *Learning disorders* (Vol. 3) (pp. 191–224). Seattle, Washington: Special Child Publications.

Denhoff, E., Davids, A., and Hawkins, R. (1971). Effects of dextroamphetamine on hyperkinetic children: A controlled double-blind study. *Journal of Learning Disabilities, 4,* 491–498.

Esterson, S. (1986). Physical therapy. In M. Esterson and L. Bluth (Eds.), *Related services for handicapped children* (pp. 79–87). Boston: Little, Brown and Company.

Exner, C. (1986). Occupational therapy. In M. Esterson and L. Bluth (Eds.), *Related services for handicapped children* (pp. 53–68). Boston: Little, Brown and Company.

Fewell, R.R., and Langley, M.B. (1984). *Developmental activities screening inventory* (DASI-II). Austin, Texas: Pro-Ed.

Firestone, P. (1982). Factors associated with children's adherence to stimulant medication. *American Journal of Orthopsychiatry, 52*(3), 447–457.

Flintoff, M.M., Barron, R.W., Swanson, J.M., Ledlow, A., and Kinsbourne, M. (1982). Methylphenidate increases selectivity of visual scanning in children referred for hyperactivity. *Journal of Abnormal Child Psychology, 10*(2), 145–161.

Gadow, K.D. (1981). *Psychosocial aspects of drug treatment for hyperactivity.* Boulder, Colorado: Westview Press.

Gittleman-Klein, R., Klein, D., Abikoff, H., Katz, S., Gloisten, A., and Kates, W. (1976). Relative efficacy of methylphenidate and behavior modification in hyperkinetic children: An interim report. *Journal of Abnormal Child Psychology, 4*(4), 361–378.

Kaufman, A., and Kaufman, N. (1983). *Kaufman assessment battery for children.* Circle Pines, Minnesota: American Guidance Service.

Kavale, K. (1982). The efficacy of drug treatment for hyperactivity: A meta-analysis. *Journal of Learning Disabilities, 15*(5), 280–289.

Lemay, D.W., Griffin, P., and Sanford, A. (1977). *Learning accomplishment profile.* Winston-Salem, North Carolina: Kaplan Press.

Loney, J. (1979). Comparing psychological and pharmacological treatments for hyperkinetic boys and their classmates. *Journal of Abnormal Child Psychology, 7*, 133–143.

Nihira, K., Foster, R., Shellhaas, M., and Leland, H. (1975). *AAMD Adaptive Behavior Scale.* San Antonio, Texas: The Psychological Corporation.

Nirje, B. (1969). The normalization principle and its human management implications. In R. Kugel and W. Wolfensberger (Eds.), *Changing patterns in residential services for the mentally retarded* (pp. 179–195). Washington, DC: United States Government Printing Office.

Pommer, L.T., Mark, D.S., and Hayden, D.L. (1983). Using computer software to instruct learning disabled students. *Learning Disabilities, 2*(8), 99–110.

Rosen, M., Clark, G., and Kivitz, M. (1977). *Habilitation of the handicapped: New dimensions in programs for the developmentally disabled.* Baltimore: University Park Press.

Shepard, L. (1983). The role of measurement in educational policy: Lessons from the identification of learning disabilities. *Educational Measurement: Issues and Practices, 2*(1), 4–8.

Sleator, E.K., Ullman, R.K., and von Neumann, A. (1982). How do hyperactive children feel about taking stimulants and will they tell the doctor? *Clinical Pediatrics, 21*, 474–479.

Sparrow, S.S., Balla, D.A., and Cicchetti, D.V. (1984). *Vineland adaptive behavior scales.* Circle Pines, Minnesota: American Guidance Services.

Sprague, R.L., and Sleator, E.K. (1977). Methylphenidate in hyperactive children: Differences in dose effects on learning and social behavior. *Science, 198*, 1274–1276.

Sykes, D., Douglas, V., and Morgenstern, G. (1972). The effect of methylphenidate (Ritalin) on sustained attention in hyperactive children. *Psychopharmacologia, 25*, 262–274.

Thorndike, R., Hagen, E., and Sattler, J. (1986). *Stanford-Binet intelligence scale—fourth revision*. Boston: Houghton Mifflin.

U.S. Department of Education. (1985). *1985 annual report to Congress on the implementation of the Education of the Handicapped Act*. Washington, DC: Government Printing Office.

U.S. Office of Education. (1977). Assistance to states for education for handicapped children: Procedure for evaluating specific learning disabilities. *Federal Register, 42*(250), 62082–62085.

Wechsler, D. (1974). *Wechsler intelligence scale for children—revised*. San Antonio, Texas: The Psychological Corporation.

Wechsler, D. (1967). *Wechsler preschool and primary scale of intelligence*. San Antonio, Texas: The Psychological Corporation.

Wender, P., and Wender, E. (1978). *The hyperactive and the learning disabled child*. New York: Crown Publishers.

Woodcock, R.W., and Johnson, M.B. (1977). *Woodcock-Johnson Psycho-Educational Battery*. Allen, Texas: Teaching Resources.

CHAPTER 7

THE EDUCATION OF CHILDREN AND ADOLESCENTS SEVERELY HANDICAPPED BY PERVASIVE DEVELOPMENTAL DISORDERS

Elaine Heffner

The education of children severely handicapped by pervasive developmental disorders increasingly has come to serve a dual function. On the one hand, it is part of a broad social mandate to educate all handicapped persons so that they may achieve their full potential. On the other hand, because there is no medical cure for these disorders, and because the impairments characteristic of these disorders interfere with usual learning, education has gone beyond usual teaching and has become a mode of therapeutic intervention. Educational interventions, therefore, have been influenced not only by general education principles adapted to the needs of this population but also by special approaches that focus on specific characteristics of the disorder as key deficits requiring treatment or remediation.

AIMS OF EDUCATION

There is considerable agreement about the broad aims of education for children with developmental handicaps. These aims are to overcome or improve primary disabilities, to prevent or ameliorate secondary handicaps, to find ways of circumventing or compensating for primary disabilities, and to teach practical skills (Callias, 1978; Rutter, 1970; Wing,

1976). Wing includes the aim of helping the handicapped person to derive as much satisfaction and enjoyment from life as possible. The first two of these aims reflect one aspect of the dual function just described, suggesting as they do a remedial focus. From an educational vantage point, the aim might be rephrased as that of teaching an appropriate curriculum to children whose learning is impaired by their disabilities. Such a statement of the goal requires further consideration of what constitutes an appropriate curriculum, the nature of the disabilities, how the disabilities impinge on learning, and what teaching methods may be useful in addressing these impediments to learning.

FACTORS INFLUENCING AIMS OF EDUCATION

The approach to these questions in specific educational programs varies in accordance with a number of factors. These include (1) the age and developmental stage of the population served, (2) the severity of the disorders addressed, and (3) the theoretical frame of reference followed. Age and stage factors are significant in distinguishing programs for the preschool and adolescent years. Particular developmental tasks are preeminent, such as the need to develop self-help skills in the preschool years and the need for vocational training in adolescence. Issues such as independent functioning have specific characteristics at these developmental stages, which must be approached differently.

The severity of the handicaps strongly influences the nature of the intervention by defining its scope, emphasis, and techniques used. For example, children who are severely impaired intellectually require different kinds of programming than those who are able to master academic tasks. Goals may be limited to improving self-care and capitalizing on any other isolated skills that may be adaptive. Extreme self-abusive or socially disruptive behavior may give rise to special approaches, such as behavioral techniques.

Differences in theoretical orientation have played an important role in shaping educational interventions. The social, behavioral, cognitive, and language deficits characteristic of pervasive developmental disorders have alternately been understood as symptoms of psychosis rooted in the early mother-child relationship or as manifestations of an abnormality of development attributable to a central nervous system disorder. These views have been translated into what may be described loosely as three models of intervention: psychoanalytic, behavioral, and developmental. Although the psychoanalytic model as such does not at present play a major role in educational interventions, psychoanalytic concepts are basic to much educational thinking, and methods from all models can be found to overlap.

MODELS OF INTERVENTION

Psychoanalytic Model

The psychoanalytic approach has been identified, in particular, with the work of Bettelheim and Mahler. Bettelheim (1967) believed that autism begins with the withdrawal of the infant from inadequate mothering. Mothers with pathological personalities respond to this withdrawal with counter-withdrawal and rejection, leaving these children empty within and shy of social trust and contact. Bettelheim viewed the behaviors characteristic of autism, such as self-stimulation and insistence on sameness, as defensive mechanisms in the service of the child's attempt to maintain homeostasis in his or her psychic environment. Interventions based on these theoretical concepts attempt to establish an environment in which the child no longer needs to rely on such devices. The Orthogenic School in Chicago, directed by Bettelheim, required that children be separated from their parents and be assigned to a counselor for 1 to 3 years in order to facilitate the reestablishment of trust and autonomy. Understanding and acceptance of regressive behaviors was accompanied by the teaching of social behavior.

Mahler (1968) devised a tripartite mode of intervention that has been applied in therapeutic nursery settings. She suggested that in one form of childhood psychosis the child withdraws into autism if the symbiotic object is lost. In the tripartite intervention, mother, child, and therapist or teacher are involved together in a "corrective symbiotic experience" in which the child, by reexperiencing earlier stages of development, is enabled to reach a higher level of development. Mahler suggested that the autistic child is unable to make use of mothering. The corrective experience is designed to foster the development of the need-satisfying symbiotic relationship between child and therapist, while at the same time training the mother to assume and maintain such a relationship. After periods of corrective symbiotic experience, children accompanied by their symbiotic partners are gradually introduced into group play.

Behavioral Model

Behavioral modification has been used in educational interventions to promote changes in specific behaviors. Learning theory views development as consisting of the acquisition of behavioral repertoires and stimulus functions. Children with pervasive developmental disorders are seen as deficient in behavioral repertoires in that they do not have the adaptive behavior that would enable them to function in society. Programs for such children may focus on strengthening certain behaviors, such as appropriate play, social interaction, and speech, by reinforcing their occurrence, or prompting and gradually shaping such behaviors by rewarding successive approximations to their final form (Lovaas, Young, and Newsom, 1978). Behavioral techniques are also used to decrease negative behavior patterns, such as tantrums, self-destructive behavior, and self-stimulation. These techniques include extinction (withholding the reinforcers that maintain them), time out (removing the child to a place where no reinforcements can be obtained), or punishment (applying aversive stimuli contingent on the occurrence of such behaviors). Food is often used as an initial reward to reinforce desired behaviors but may, in time, be replaced by external praise and ultimately by the child's own self-praise or inner control.

Although some programs follow a behavioral orientation in their approach to all learning, behavioral techniques are also used within other types of interventions to address specific deficits. In particular, behavioral techniques have been used to eliminate self-destructive and self-stimulative behavior and to address the problems of delayed and deviant language. Although success has been reported both in eliminating deviant behavior and in teaching receptive and expressive language (Lovaas *et al.*, 1978), a number of problems have been noted: an increase in lexicon without increase in linguistic complexity, and, in particular, poor generalization from the learning environment to other situations. Lovaas and colleagues attribute this to the use of artificial reinforcers, such as food, in the absence of knowledge about motivational factors or normal reinforcers. Gains have been maintained more effectively when parents are trained to continue the behavioral program at home, and parent training is an important component of behavioral interventions. Another limitation of these methods is that they require sustained effort on a one-to-one basis. Behavioral interventions are discussed in more detail in Chapter 5.

Developmental Model

The developmental approach looks at both deficits and behavior in terms of deviance and delays within a developmental frame. Schopler (1976) pointed out that children's adaptational skills and the manifestations of their handicaps are formed, in part, by their age and developmental level. Characteristic of these disorders is a range of developmental levels in the various skills and behaviors of individual children. In addition, the level of intelligence and the degree and extent of impairment are not the same for all children. Individual differences may be more relevant than similarities within diagnostic categories.

Educational programs, rather than focusing on deficits per se, seek to determine the educational implications of these deficits for the individual child based on his or her developmental level in significant areas of functioning. Assessment is made of areas of strength and weakness, which becomes the basis of an individualized educational plan (IEP) within the context of a group program.

In general, IEPs draw from a knowledge of normal development with a focus on tasks that are within a child's abilities and have relevance to his or her daily life. Language, reading and number concepts, self-help skills, and behaviors that interfere with learning are among the content areas included in educational programs. A variety of techniques taken from regular education, special education, and behavioral approaches have been used to address perceptual-motor and cognitive deficits, but these must be adapted to the individual child's learning patterns. Lansing and Schopler (1978) pointed to the pressures operating against individualized curricula, which include too many children and too few teachers and classes, lack of adequate training for teachers in individualizing curricula, administrative pressures to use one teaching system to the exclusion of others, and inadequate communication with parents to facilitate transfer from classroom to home and back. In part because of these pressures, there is great diversity among programs and in interpretations of the meaning of following a developmental approach. The intended focus on the child may shift to a focus on deficits, and an emphasis on special techniques may substitute for a knowledge of the child's own learning pattern.

GENERAL ISSUES IN CHOOSING AN INTERVENTION

The translation of broad educational aims into specific curriculum content and teaching methods is influenced by the child's age and developmental stage, the severity of the disorder, and the theoretical orientation of involved professionals. Other questions must also be considered by educational interventions. One of these relates to the classification and grouping of children. As described earlier, atypical behavior can occur in association with any level of intelligence, and an extreme range of functioning may be found in children who fall within the same psychiatric diagnosis. This points to grouping on the basis of children's specific impairments and level of functioning, rather than on the basis of diagnostic categories. Wing and Wing (1976) pointed out that specialized services, to be organized in such a manner, have to draw from large populations, and this may not be a viable approach in many communities. Attempts to fit children with these disorders into classes of children with other handicaps may also be a problem because of the specific adaptation of teaching methods and special understanding required for this population. Finally, there is a mandate to provide the "least restrictive environment," which means balancing a child's optimal level of functioning with his or her need for special intervention and individualized approaches.

Another general question concerns whether and how parents are to be integrated into the educational program. All theoretical approaches agree on the importance of work with parents. Schopler (1976) points out that the directions of a young child's development are based on the interactions with his or her parents. Normally, parents tend to gear their expectations to a child's age and developmental level. The atypical development and behavior of children with pervasive developmental disorders confuses and worries parents, affecting their behavior with their children. Parents need help with confusions about their children's difficulties and with erroneous expectations. They need to become more effective in their management of children at home and in fulfilling their long-term responsibility to obtain appropriate services for their children. Beyond that, much of the educational work that has been done has demonstrated the importance of parent involvement in generalizing and maintaining children's gains. In various programs, parents are worked with individually or in groups, receiving advice, counseling or psychotherapy. They have been trained to work with teachers and children in the classroom, to function as cotherapists, and to carry out behavioral programs in the home. Typically, preschool programs have more significant parent components than do programs for school-age children, although there is a general consensus that on-going work with parents is desirable.

In addition to these general issues—how best to group children and how to involve parents—and to the factors discussed earlier that influence educational interventions—the child's age and developmental stage, the severity of the disorder, and the preferred theoretical frame of reference—there are specific educational principles related to curriculum and methods that are generally applied but that are interpreted in a variety of ways in existing programs. These will be discussed in the sections that follow on preschool and school-age educational interventions.

THERAPEUTIC NURSERIES

The therapeutic nursery, at present the primary mode of intervention for preschool children severely handicapped by developmental disorders, reflects the joining of theories and practices of both education and psychiatry. Growing out of work with displaced children separated from their families during World Wars I and II, and using educational methods based on psychoanalytic techniques, therapeutic nurseries were extended to serve children with emotional problems and later to children with retardation, deviance, and severe mental illness (Shapiro and Sherman, 1984). A general emphasis on early intervention developed in the 1960s in the wake of research pointing to the importance of early stimulation to later academic success. In addition, within psychiatry, changing views of the developmental disorders shifted the focus from attempts at cure to remediation, and, therefore, to educational interventions. Finally, the mandating of education for all handicapped children was extended to the preschool population as well.

In some ways the therapeutic nursery serves the same function for the developmentally handicapped child as it does for the normal child: It introduces him or her to a school routine, to separation from his or her parents, to interactions with teachers and peers, to the use of materials, and to the rules of social living. Such exposure is, if anything, more essential for the handicapped child whose impairments mean that a much longer time will be required before he or she can participate in and learn from these experiences.

Deficits in Early Childhood

Rutter (1979) suggested that the three chief handicaps of autism are (1) the failure of social development, particularly the failure to develop early normal attachment behavior; (2) failure of language development; and (3) the tendency to develop rigid, stereotypic, ritualistic behaviors. These failures, deviations, and delays in development that characterize pervasive developmental disorders are manifest in the first years of life. This means that the usual learning that takes place in early childhood is interrupted and that children with these disorders soon become functionally retarded. When children fail to develop normal attachment behavior, the relationship with the mother (or caregiver)—the primary source of learning about the social world—is unavailable as a stimulus to the development of social behavior and as a bridge to the larger social world. The absence of language and the broadening impairment of communication skills act to cut the child off still further from the usual learning experiences of the preschool years. Likewise, rigidities and ritualistic behaviors serve to reinforce the child's isolation and to interfere with the usual interactions that promote learning and contribute to development. It is often difficult to determine where primary disabilities end and secondary deficits, stemming from the breakdown of learning in the first years of life, begin. Early intervention of an educational nature, therefore, has twofold importance: (1) It serves a corrective function by promoting learning that in normal development would occur in more natural ways, and (2) it has a diagnostic function by determining a child's capacity for learning and growth, thereby making possible more accurate assessment of underlying deficits.

Although therapeutic nurseries vary in accordance with the different theoretical orientations discussed earlier, they share the goals of overcoming or improving primary disabilities and of intervening in secondary deficits and behavior problems. These goals have particular relevance for the preschool years because they are a time of maximum maturational and developmental spurts, which can be enlisted in the service of an educational intervention. Moreover, secondary behaviors and deficits may not yet be so deeply entrenched and, therefore, may be more amenable to intervention. Normally these years are the time for the acquisition of many skills (social, cognitive, and physical), which serve as a base for later development, thus making it critical that emerging disabilities be addressed as they are unfolding. Finally, primary disabilities are not yet as fully compounded as they will be later in a child increasingly cut off from usual learning experiences.

The Effect of Pervasive Developmental Disorders on Learning

Using a developmental model, Rutter and Sussenwein (1971) focused on failures in social and language development and on the tendency toward rigid, stereotyped, or ritualistic behavior. They sought to identify the ways in which disordered development departed from normality, to determine the defects that led to this departure, to consider what was required for normal development, and then to determine what had to be provided for a more normal development. Failures in social development begin in the earliest mother-child interactions. At the extreme end of the spectrum of disorders, infants appear unresponsive to social stimuli, do not make normal eye contact, and fail to develop a social smile or to reach out to be picked up. The infant exhibits few or none of the behaviors that parents normally interpret as wanting or needing attention, and consequently parental response and interaction with the infant is greatly diminished. Whatever the primary disability, it is compounded by the lack of social stimulation. Beyond that, however, with few clear "requests" for attention, parents are less likely to become successful providers of relief from distress or to adequately meet the needs of the infant. All of these factors interfere with the development of attachment behavior and bonds, which are the basis for later social development. Typical preverbal communication patterns between mother and child fail to develop. Consequently children do not have the experience of having an effect on their environment, of learning that communication of needs can result in gratification. Deprivation sustained in this area has implications for the development of more sophisticated communication skills later on. In general, a primary deficit in the ability to elicit responses from the social world results in an absence of the experiences that promote development; interactions with the environment in which learning usually takes place do not occur or are skewed. As a result, not only are children impaired in their ability to relate to others but they also fail to develop age-appropriate skills.

Functioning at Time of Referral

Referral to a therapeutic nursery usually occurs when children are between 2 and 4 years of age. Often, at the time of referral, they still drink from a bottle and are not toilet trained. They have few self-help skills and are perceived and treated by their parents as if they are much younger than their chronological ages. Parents are typically confused about the child's level of competence and fail to set appropriate expectations or teach appropriate skills. This serves to reinforce primary deficits. Often these children show little interest in other adults or children and appear not to expect adults to be a source of pleasure or of understanding and fulfillment of needs. When they do approach others, they do so in unacceptable and unsuccessful ways, often using behaviors that appear aggressive or are typical of the social approaches of a younger child, such as hair pulling, biting, pushing. Likewise, their responses to others may be atypical, such as tuning out approaches made to them or striking out when approached.

Frequently these children have no language or delayed or atypical language skills, and they do not use language to communicate effectively or to interact successfully with others. Because of these children's unresponsiveness, deficits in receptive language, and poor communicative skills, parents are confused about their children's level of comprehension. Parents often stop using language with these children and feel there is no way to teach them or to convey expectations. Once again, primary deficits serve to close off interactions with the environment, thereby interrupting the usual learning process, intensifying primary disabilities, and creating secondary deficits.

Children are most often behind age level in areas of general information, grasp of concepts involving time, space, and social relationships, and sequential thinking. It may be difficult to determine, initially, the degree to which these delays reflect primary disabilities or secondary deficits. In these areas, intervention serves a strong diagnostic function.

Goals and Methods of Intervention in the Therapeutic Nursery

Translating this view of pervasive developmental disorders into specific educational approaches means finding ways of providing the experiences that are usually part of early childhood learning to children who are not learning in usual ways. This suggests both adapting the curriculum of the normal nursery school to the needs and skill levels of these children and finding methods by which individual children may be helped to make use of the curriculum that is provided. As discussed earlier, the failure to develop social contact and the consequent impairment of interactions with parents interfere with the earliest learning experiences, and this impairment remains a primary obstacle to learning. The first goal, therefore, is to establish communication between teacher and child as an avenue for learning and for entering a larger social world.

Several aspects must be considered in working toward this goal. The first is that these children, to a great extent, have not experienced adults as potentially need-gratifying objects or as sources of pleasure. The teacher must find ways to create these experiences. Children's behavior, which is sometimes viewed as a separate issue, is actually highly relevant in this regard. Because these children are impaired in communication skills, behavior such as tantrums, crying, tuning out, and even stereotypic movements may be their only way of expressing needs and wants or of responding to situations experienced as stressful. For example, it has been found both in clinical observation and experimentally that these behaviors occur when children are given tasks that are too difficult for them to perform (Wing, 1976). Through careful monitoring of the context in which behavior occurs, it is often possible to discern the communicative function the behavior serves for the child, albeit most often a negative function, as such behavior typically elicits negative responses from the environment.

Careful observation of children's behavior is important in other ways as well. Positive responses may be as difficult to spot as the meaning of negative behavior is to interpret, and it is only through close attention that the child's flickers of interest in materials or events may be discerned. It is possible, then, to build experiences on these initial minimal responses, experiences which children will find pleasurable and which will, therefore, engage them. In this way, the teacher not only becomes the source of pleasurable experiences for the child, thereby contributing to the development of a relationship between them, but is also in a position to widen the areas of experience necessary for learning.

Observation also plays a significant role in identifying the levels at which children are functioning in various areas of development. This information is critical in providing experiences for children in which they can be successful. Because these children's impairments make it difficult for them to meet the ordinary demands of living and the expectations of their parents, the experience of failure is the perpetual condition of their lives (Wing, 1976). Many of them have had virtually no experience of the pleasure that comes with success. To provide such success experiences, it is necessary first to know the level at which a child is able to perform, so that the tasks provided are ones at which the child will be competent and, therefore, successful. It is through such success that children develop the positive attitudes toward learning that enable them to approach new skills, materials, and experiences. The child can then be led on with praise and support for his or her achievements. Activities that do not have a clearly built-in teacher goal as the measure of a child's success make it possible to follow the child's own ideas and interests, which further increases his or her confidence.

The relationship with the teacher can also help to move children into peer interactions and the rewards of social experiences. Successful social interactions require the communication skills that are a major area of impairment in these children. Rutter (1979) notes the importance of developing prelinguistic skills and language comprehension through play, the encouragement of imitative behavior, and the introduction of talking into the play situation in a way that is linked with what the child or adult is doing. He indicates that the objective is communication rather than speech as such and suggests that it is desirable to encourage the child's communications in whatever form they appear, with a particular emphasis on the social components of communication. As discussed earlier, children with pervasive developmental disorders most often have not had the usual experiences in preverbal communication with parents, as parents are unable to understand and, therefore, respond to absent or unclear signals. As also stated earlier, these children do not have the experience of having an effect on the environment through communication which, in normal development, motivates further attempts at communication. To create successful social interactions, these children must first be given experiences that demonstrate to them that it is possible for them to make themselves understood and that it is rewarding to try. Teachers can accomplish this by working to understand and respond to a child's nonverbal or behavioral communication. In this regard, work with parents can be a significant component of an educational intervention because when parents are helped to understand the behavioral communications of their children, they not only become more effective in meeting their needs, they also facilitate expanding efforts at communication on the part of their children.

DEVELOPMENTAL MODEL THERAPEUTIC NURSERY

To demonstrate the ways in which the foregoing concepts are applied in an educational intervention, the therapeutic nursery at Payne Whitney Clinic, New York Hospital, will be described. This program is part of the section on child psychiatry and is housed in a large medical center. The nursery space includes adjoining rooms for children and parents, separated by a one-way screen and an open door that allows easy access from one room to another. Children are referred from pediatric clinics, private physicians, other educational or therapeutic facilities, and direction centers set up throughout the city to direct families of handicapped children to appropriate resources. The program accepts children who are between 2 and 5 years of age and who are delayed or deviant in development.

Assessment of Developmentally Disordered Children

Parents and children are seen in an initial screening interview conducted in the nursery by a social worker, a psychiatrist, and a teacher-therapist who is trained in early childhood special education. The educational evaluation is not a formal testing situation. Instead, the teacher explores the child's range of functioning using the materials and activities of the nursery setting, as well as his or her knowledge of the wide variety of ways in which young children learn from and interact with their environment. The dolls, books, soap suds, wagons, games, and people of the nursery become the equipment for measuring development. The teacher's concern, for example, is not to find out if the child can build a three block tower, but to see exactly how he or she uses the blocks; does he bang them, throw them, line them up, explore them with eyes, fingers, mouth, build a garage, or turn away uninterested? The teacher tries to connect to a child at his or her various developmental levels, to expand his play, his language, his physical skills, finding out what he or she can teach and the child can learn. In this way the teacher assesses physical, cognitive, social, and emotional development, paying special attention to the emotional needs of children whose self-esteem and sense of self have often been badly marred and retarded by their failure to learn in the usual ways or at the usual pace (Balliett, 1978).

As the teacher is engaging the child, the social worker interviews the parents. This, too, is less a formal history-taking session than an attempt to learn the parents' view of the problem, their perceptions of the child's behavior, mode of interacting with the child, emotional state with regard to the child's impairment, and readiness to become engaged in a therapeutic program. When the teacher appears to have engaged the child on some level, the parents are led by the social worker to an adjoining room to make some assessment of how both child and parents deal with separation. The psychiatrist may continue the observation of the child with the teacher, may join the discussion with the parents, or may alternate between the two rooms. The psychiatrist may also seek more medical and developmental information from the parents.

Following this initial screening interview, the members of the team meet to discuss their observations and to formulate a recommendation for disposition. If the recommendation is that the child be accepted into the nursery program, a determination is also made about the appropriate group assignment based on the existing composition of the groups and the initial appraisal of the child's current level of functioning and educational needs. Assignment is also made to a child psychiatrist, who will do a more complete individual evaluation and will serve as the child's physician during his or her time in the nursery program. A more formal developmental evaluation is also done by a psychologist, who then functions as a member of the on-going team.

Operation of the Program

The therapeutic nursery generally serves 10 to 12 children in two groups that meet for $2\frac{1}{2}$ hours a day. Frequency of attendance is determined according to the needs of the individual child. Children are also seen individually once a week so that the teacher-therapist can work with them more intensively on the areas of difficulty that have been observed in the nursery setting. A group of five to six children has two teacher-therapists and often a student or aide assisting as well. The parents of each group meet once a week in the adjoining room while the nursery is in session. These groups are led by a psychiatrist or social worker. The psychiatrists who follow the individual children observe them on a regular basis in the nursery and, when indicated, recommend additional tests or procedures that may be useful in determining causes of disorders. Psychiatrists also meet with the parents individually if necessary. Team meetings held once a week are used to review the progress of each group of children and parents, and periodic case conferences focus more fully on each family.

A great deal of attention is given to the composition of the groups of children in the nursery. Whenever possible, the groups are heterogeneous with regard to behavior, developmental deficits, and strengths. Most children do not present a classic prototype of a particular diagnostic category, but rather cover a broad developmental spectrum of delays, deviance, and behavior, with different combinations of high and low levels of functioning in individual children. Such differences may be useful within the group. For example, children who are extremely active or aggressive may attract the attention of those who are more withdrawn or passive. Children who use language may provide a model for those who do not. It is not unusual for a child to engage the interest of other children in ways that can then be used by the teacher to facilitate social interactions. On the other hand, an effort is made to provide children with some peers who can match their level of functioning.

Goals of the Program

There are three goals for the children in the nursery program. The first goal is diagnostic clarification. As discussed earlier, secondary disabilities and behavioral difficulties may compound primary deficits, clouding the true picture of a child's capacity for growth and development. During the course of intervention, change or its absence permits a more accurate assessment of a child's potential. The entire period of the child's attendance in the nursery is viewed as an extended evaluation that will provide a fuller understanding of his or her range of functioning and make possible more accurate planning for future educational and therapeutic needs.

The second goal of the nursery is to provide the educational experiences that are usually part of early childhood learning and development. This means facilitating trusting relationships with other adults, play and learning interactions with peers, and explorations of the physical environment through the use of the senses.

The third goal is to improve functioning in language and communication skills and in emotional, social, cognitive, and physical development. To accomplish this requires both a detailed knowledge of each child's capacities and limitations and careful planning of activities so that children are given tasks at which they can be successful. As the emphasis is not on one-to-one relationships but on moving children into peer interactions and the rewards of social experiences, it is necessary to devise activities that make possible children's participation at varying levels of competence. Particularly desirable are activities that can be used to address many aspects of development at different levels of development. For example, an activity such as the water table can serve many functions simultaneously: at the most basic sensory-motor level, children can simply trail their hands in the water or splash; on the symbolic, representational level of dramatic play, they can sail boats or give the dolls a bath; at the cognitive level, concepts such as full, empty, or sinking can be introduced; at the fine motor level, children can open and close caps of water bottles or squeeze spray bottles. As a social activity, children can participate on the level of parallel play, engage in interactive games, or be helped to take turns with the water toys. As with other activities, for some children participation may mean just watching. Because of the range of possibilities within the activity, children are able to participate successfully at their own levels. Motor activities, such as the slide, similarly enable children to come together without requiring a specific level of skill, at the same time opening possibilities to try the next steps when they are ready.

The use of language is an important component in all of the activities of the nursery. The teacher uses language to clarify experiences, simplify concepts, highlight key aspects of events, and provide words or phrases that can work for children as they attempt to gratify their wants or needs. Repetition is important in all use of language. The teacher also uses language as a social bridge, often narrating aloud the events of the nursery room and helping to make children aware of each other by describing what each one is doing. In this way, a social connection can be made even when children are physically in separate corners of the room.

Promotion of Communication

The children in the program are impaired not only in language skills but also in other areas of functioning necessary for the development of communication skills, such as appropriate contact with the environment and attention focusing. A fundamental goal of the educational program, therefore, is to provide the experiences that will promote communication or successful interactions with others. To accomplish this, communication must first be established between teachers and children, which means children must be allowed to communicate in whatever ways are available to them. In one sense, all behavior can be viewed as a form of communication, although one that may require observation and knowledge of the individual child to be understood. Because of their many experiences of failure and the absence of pleasurable interactions with others, children often express their negative feelings in unacceptable and self-defeating behavior. To interrupt the cycle of children's negative behavior eliciting negative responses from the environment, teachers begin by responding first to the communicative meaning of the behavior rather than to the negative form in which it is expressed. By responding to the communication first, rather than focusing first on the behavior, the teacher in effect gives the children permission to let him or her know what their needs and feelings are in any way that they can. Accepting the child's communication does not mean that the teacher condones the child's behavior or way of communicating. Once a child learns to trust the teacher as one who is responsive to his or her needs, the child can then learn from the teacher other, more acceptable ways of making himself or herself understood (Balliett and Heffner, 1974; Heffner and Balliett, 1976).

Because a child's first experience with communication is in the mother-child relationship, a major emphasis is placed on understanding mother-child interactions. This focus makes it possible to identify the ways in which mother and child are missing each other in their communications. When children express their needs and wishes in ways that are not age-appropriate, the responses of the mothers are also inappropriate. The atypical development of the children leads to inaccurate perceptions by parents of children's deficits, areas of competence, and the meaning of their behavior. These perceptions, as well as disturbed feelings about having atypical children, interfere with the ability of parents to respond to children in ways that are nurturing and to set appropriate expectations. Both perceptions and feelings must be addressed in the work with parents. Specifically, parents need help in understanding the behavioral communications of their children in a developmental context. In one sense, the intervention is focused on reopening communication between mother and child by providing for each of them the ingredient that is missing in their relationship with each other. For the mother, this means an experience in understanding what a child is saying through behavior: the child's behavior is made intelligible to her. For the child it means an experience in successful preverbal communication: an experience with someone who understands and responds to what is communicated by his or her behavior.

The case material that follows is illustrative of work with a severely handicapped child in the therapeutic nursery.

Jack was 4 years old when referred to the nursery because of his failure to develop language, his lack of social relatedness, and many stereotypic behaviors, such as looking at his hands and laughing to himself while running back and forth. During psychiatric examination he avoided eye contact, did not follow any commands, made a variety of unintelligible sounds, and spoke no words. He did not play reciprocally and, in general, just shook or threw various toys to the floor. During psychological evaluation he wandered about, stood by the door making distressed sounds, jumped on the test materials, and pinched the skin on top of his mother's hand. In the initial nursery evaluation the teacher-therapist noted that his running around the room "seemed to be his way of exploring." She was successful at engaging him in three activities: after bouncing a ball and handing it to him he looked at her with good eye contact, dropped the ball, and waited for her to do it again. He also stayed close by a bubble blowing activity and popped a bubble after the teacher popped one. Later, he allowed the teacher to help him use the slide successfully. It was her impression that although he was very difficult to engage, he did relate to her and to the materials in an oblique way.

This oblique style was found to characterize Jack's approach to all of the activities of the nursery school. In the initial phase he did a great deal of running back and forth in the room. The teacher joined him in his running and invented running games, which other children sometimes joined. Gradually, his running decreased and the teachers noticed that he would hover on the fringes of an activity and spend time indirectly watching out of the corner of his eye. They found that at these times he was more open to taking the risk of reaching out and touching materials. His watching became the first step in leading him into the activity itself, with both interest and use of materials developing at the sensory-motor level (bubbles, water play, and musical instruments). The teachers helped him take the step from observation to participation by encouraging and supporting an entry level of participation, which for him was often knocking something down to the floor. Next, he was helped to use an object in a more explorative fashion such as banging, shaking, or visually examining it. Through close observation the teachers began to understand his indirect communications. For example, when he wanted to use the climber he would go over and stand next to it. At these times the teacher could provide what he wanted while expressing to him, in words, her understanding of the situation. At other times, however, when his needs were not understood, he became very agitated and would bite and scratch. Here the teacher provided physical and verbal support, expressing in simple language her recognition of his feelings, her wish to help him, and her assurance that she would not permit him to hurt himself or her.

Jack's approach to other children followed the indirect style he used with materials. Initially, he spent time watching the other children. Next, he would stand close to them and finally began taking their hands, trying to have them come and play with him. If another child rebuffed his invitation to play, he was often torn between continuing or abandoning an activity. Here the teacher provided clarification and support to create successful interactions with other children whenever possible, assisting him in taking turns, and focusing his attention on where he was, what he was doing, where the other children were, and what they were doing.

Jack especially enjoyed gross motor activities and was agile and competent at climbing, jumping, and sliding. After a long period of watching, he began to imitate some of the other children's various ways of sliding and climbing. He enjoyed sitting next to another child at the top of the climber. He also began to participate in fine motor activites (peg board, stickers, beating on a drum, and pouring liquids into a cup), which initially he had avoided.

Jack was able to feed himself, independently use the bathroom, help dress and undress himself, and go to his mother for emotional support. Another asset was his good memory; he would take a teacher to a locked cabinet, looking for a specific piece of equipment that was used the day before. He came to form expectations about school, anticipating and asking for activities, such as climbing, snack, and water play. Although he did not develop expressive language, his receptive language improved, particularly when language was combined with an activity or toy. His communication became more direct, and he actively brought the teacher to the material or activity that he wanted.

During Jack's time in the nursery his mother attended a mothers' group. Two issues relating to her interactions with Jack assumed special significance. Because of his lack of language and indirect way of relating, she had come to believe that he had no special attachment to her and that her presence or absence was of little consequence to him. During group sessions he would, as other children did, come back to where the mothers were meeting to see her and would stand somewhat behind her chair and to the side. She never greeted him and either ignored his presence completely or angrily pushed him back into the nursery room. She would often arrive back with her hands scratched, as if she had been attacked by a cat. She revealed that this was caused by Jack's scratching and pinching, which she did nothing about, believing that there was nothing she could do. Basically, Jack's mother believed there was no way to have effective communication between Jack and herself in either direction. These issues were worked on in the group, with other mothers expressing the view that it was obvious to them that Jack was attached to her and was actually coming back to see her rather than to disobediently leave the nursery room, as she believed. Gradually, she began to give him positive responses, to which he clearly reacted with pleasure, until one day he spontaneously came over to her and gave her a hug. The group also worked on the scratching issue, insisting that Jack's mother not permit him to do this to her. She was given many suggestions, but the group encouragement, rather than their suggestions, enabled her to find her own method of dealing with this. The key appeared to be her gradual belief that she could have an effect on him, supported in part by her growing awareness that she was significant to him.

One year later, Jack's mother was seen in a follow-up visit and talked about her feeling that so much progress had been made despite her disappointment that he had not developed language. The meaningful areas of change she cited were in his behavioral problems, his ability to follow routines, and his increased understanding. Most of all, however, she had found that she could reach him and therefore could deal with many more situations, which had improved the quality of their family life.

SCHOOL-AGE EDUCATIONAL INTERVENTIONS

Defining an appropriate curriculum and useful teaching methods for interventions at school-age levels, as for preschool interventions, is related to the nature of children's disabilities and the ways in which these affect learning. As pointed out earlier, children's adaptational skills and the manifestations of their impairments are shaped in part by their ages and developmental levels. At the same time, the increasing complexity of academic tasks typically widens the gap between children's skills and usual school curricula. There has been some disagreement about whether to follow a normal developmental sequence in planning curriculum. Should goals be based on skills that are developmentally just ahead of a child's present level of functioning or should the sequence of normal development be disregarded? (Callias, 1978) The latter approach has been followed in some interventions directed toward specific deficits, such as those in language and perceptual skills, and toward inappropriate behaviors. The failure to generalize or maintain trained skills and behavior, however, is itself a deficit that must be considered in devising the content and methods of an educational program. Deficits in receptive and expressive language, in social interaction, and in response to environmental stimuli mean that children do not learn spontaneously. Also, they are easily overwhelmed by their own uncontrollable behavior, which increases anxiety and leads to regression and further disorganization (Fenichel, 1974).

In light of these factors, there is general agreement that children respond best to systematic teaching in a structured setting and an ordered environment (Bartak, 1978; Callias, 1978; Wing, 1976). The concept of structure, however, has been subject to differing interpretations. Bartak (1978) describes two aspects of structure: structuring the child's responses, and structuring the stimuli reaching the child. The first refers to a task orientation in which the adult determines what the child should be doing, whereas the second refers to an environment that is limited, planned, and organized. Rutter and Bartak (1973) suggested that structure should not imply rigidity, rote learning, or forcing the child to perform.

EXAMPLES OF SCHOOL AGE INTERVENTIONS

TEACCH

TEACCH, the North Carolina state program for autistic children, is based on a developmental model. It is designed to facilitate individualization and transfer to the child's daily life (Lansing and Schopler, 1978; Schopler and Reichler, 1979). Classrooms of six to eight children with a teacher and teacher aide are located in public schools and are under the direction of centers that provide counseling and teaching to individual children and their families. In the centers, parents are involved as cotherapists, working jointly with therapists to develop curricula and teaching techniques for home teaching that take into consideration the child's developmental level and the parents' priorities and resources. This home program is demonstrated in weekly sessions at the center. The same process takes place in the classroom, with an emphasis on group teaching and school routines. Parent participation in the center and the classroom facilitates transfer between the child's learning experiences at school and at home.

Assessment of children is based on a psycho-educational profile, standard intelligence tests, parent interviews, and direct observation of parent-child interactions. Using early childhood materials , such as soap bubbles and beads, the psycho-educational profile screens functioning in six areas: imitation, perception, motor behavior, eye-hand integration, and expressive and receptive language skills. Tasks at which the child is not yet successful, but shows some understanding of, are regarded as emerging skills and become the basis of the individualized home program and classroom curriculum. An appropriate curriculum is derived both from the assessment procedures, which indicate the range of the child's developmental level, and from the teacher's observations and learning trials with the individual child. In planning curriculum, activities and materials are used that are at the child's emerging level of ability and that will be familiar and useful in daily life. Tasks are designed to use a child's strengths and to provide training of deficit areas. In particular, the educational program is designed to promote growth in human relatedness, perceptual-motor organization, and cognitive functioning.

Lansing and Schopler (1978) described a controversial task analysis approach for teaching skills. Teacher and parent together select tasks that are both within the child's ability and important for daily living.

The child's interests and learning style are identified through shared observations and are taken into account in the structuring of the task. Tasks are then broken down into steps of increasing difficulty commensurate with the child's increased skill. An example is given of a buttoning task, which begins with pushing poker chips through a card, moves on to large buttons, then smaller buttons, and finally buttons attached to cloth. The concept of big and little is also taught through sorting tasks, using home and school materials. On the basis of shared observations between home and school, the child's training is expanded from specific structured tasks to many daily routines. Behavior management techniques are used in teaching and are based on the child's level of awareness and total environment. Parents participate in establishing behavioral goals and choices of rewards and punishments.

Education in Adolescence

Fredericks, Buckley, Baldwin, and Stremel-Campbell (1983) stated that the goal of education for autistic adolescents should be to help them function more independently in society and to perform more normally by reducing aberrant behaviors. They recommend that the educational environment include a focus on functional living skills, parent involvement, support services, and classroom management and teaching strategies. Education must go beyond the classroom to home, stores, restaurants, and similar environments if any level of independent functioning is to be achieved. Also, parents must be involved in carry-over of teaching into the home so that generalization of skills can occur. For example, if a student has been taught to tell time, he or she will lose that skill if not required to tell time at home. Support services such as speech or physical therapy provide additional input for teachers and parents in their work with the student.

The Teaching Research Infant and Child Center, the specific educational program described by Fredericks and colleagues (1983), includes an individualized program for each student, group and individual instruction, the use of volunteers to provide some individual instruction, attention to the remediation of inappropriate behaviors in the classroom, the incorporation of support personnel into classroom management, and checklists used to monitor the quality of instruction. Both a total task approach and a task-analyzed approach are used in teaching. The former means that a task is modeled for the student, and he or she then tries to perform it and is given feedback when difficulty occurs. A task-analyzed approach means teaching a task step by step. A variety of techniques are used to facilitate generalization to new materials, people, and settings. These include multiple exemplars (using several objects in training), selecting cues that are common to both

training setting and settings desired for generalization, concurrent training (learning more than one behavior at a time), and the gradual use
of natural consequences and indiscriminable contingencies.

The curriculum described by Fredericks and colleagues is adapted
to the individual needs of the student and includes social and sexual
skills, practical living skills, leisure time skills, vocational education,
and functional academics. Social and sexual skills include developing
social behaviors that are taught by placing the student in social situations, then role-playing or otherwise correcting the behavior through
a reinforcement or feedback system. Practical living skills include personal hygiene, care of clothing, handling money, and similar activities.
Leisure activities relate both to those at home and those in the community. The vocational program consists, first, of short-term exposure
to a number of jobs in the school, such as maintenance, food service,
or clerical. Next, the student spends 6 months in two of these settings,
the placement based on prior performance and student preference. Here
the student is taught more of the skills involved in the work. Finally,
the student is placed in a community job with training that can lead
to long-term employment. In the functional academics component of
the curriculum, the emphasis is on the practical aspect of skills, such
as the use of mathematics in handling money, use of reading to follow
directions, and so forth. In general, the curriculum includes age-
appropriate materials and activities geared to the individual student's
developmental level.

A Board of Education Model

The New York City Board of Education has established units called
Specialized Instructional Environments to serve children with pervasive
developmental disorders who are seriously handicapped. One of these
units (Manhattan) is divided into three age groupings, which are
roughly 5 to 8 years, 8 through 12 years, and 13 to 21 years. Groups
consist of five to six children, in accordance with the functional level
of the children and the legal restriction that age ranges not exceed 3
years. Each group has one teacher and one allied professional member.
General staffing also includes one speech teacher for every 20 children,
one or more adaptive physical education teachers, toilet trainers for
incontinent children, and vocational or educational specialists in the
older groups. Curriculum includes reading, language arts, mathematics,
gross and fine motor perception, speech and communicative skills,
activities of daily living, art, and prevocational and vocational skills
workshops.

The approach used is described as psychoeducational. This means
that the teacher uses a developmental assessment of the child's daily
functioning in the classroom to devise an educational program that is

functional and uses concrete materials that are within the experience of the child. The classroom is highly structured and a task-analysis approach is often used, but without behavioral techniques. Principles of positive reinforcement are used without external rewards; reinforcement is accomplished through praise or rewards in the form of activities the child enjoys. Behavior is not dealt with as such, but only as it interferes with the task at hand. Inappropriate behavior is ignored or redirected whenever possible. Within the classroom, the teacher may work with two or three children at a time while the assistant works with the others. Tasks are teacher-directed, with a strong emphasis on keeping the child's focus on the teacher and maintaining attention until a task is complete. A total communication approach is used, which includes signing as well as spoken language. A major goal of this program is to develop independent functioning to the degree possible for the individual child, and to this end a variety of techniques are used to promote generalization. An interesting aspect of this model is its affiliation with the Association in Manhattan for Autistic Children. This voluntary association of parents provides auxiliary services, such as psychiatric consultation and after-school and summer programs.

SUMMARY

Despite the many variations in educational interventions that result from differences in theoretical orientation, interpretations of concepts, and teaching styles, shared underlying principles in these educational interventions can also be identified. In general, educational programs seek to fulfill the dual purpose of educating children to the extent of their potential, while at the same time providing remediation or therapy for the handicaps that characterize their disorders. Some interventions have focused on addressing the deficits themselves, whereas others seek to overcome or circumvent handicaps as they interfere with achieving broader goals. The content of curriculum changes with the age and developmental stage of the population involved, but there is general recognition of the need to individualize goals and content according to the range of functioning and the strengths and deficits of the particular child. Such knowledge of the child is derived from various assessment measures and also from observation over time. All programs seek to strengthen social, communicative, and cognitive skills and to address atypical behavior. Behavioral techniques and special education techniques have been used and at times overused in an attempt to make them applicable to all children.

Schopler and Mesibov (1985) suggested that just as there was a shift at an earlier time from speech and operant therapies to language therapy, a shift is now taking place from language therapy to communication training. This means less emphasis on one-to-one teaching of specific words and more emphasis on tying communication training to a child's specific interests and activities and on alternative communication systems. The same trend can be observed in other areas of curriculum content, which increasingly are designed to provide experiences and learning that have relevance to the child in his or her world. Finally, there is a general recognition of the importance of involving parents in educational programs, not only to achieve immediate goals with children but also to sustain parents in their difficult task of raising severely handicapped children.

REFERENCES

Balliett, E. (1978). Teacher evaluations of preschool children with developmental problems. *Special Children, 4*, 35–41.

Balliett, E., and Heffner, E. (1974). *Program report, Nursery School Treatment Center.* Unpublished manuscript, Payne Whitney Clinic, New York, New York.

Bartak, L. (1978). Educational approaches. In M. Rutter and E. Schopler (Eds.), *Autism: A reappraisal of concepts and treatment* (pp. 423–432). New York: Plenum Press.

Bettelheim, B. (1967). *The empty fortress.* New York: The Free Press.

Callias, M. (1978). Educational aims and methods. In M. Rutter and E. Schopler (Eds.), *Autism: A reappraisal of concepts and treatment* (pp. 453–461). New York: Plenum Press.

Fenichel, C. (1974). Special education as the basic therapeutic tool in treatment of severely disturbed children. *Journal of Autism and Childhood Schizophrenia, 4*, 177–186.

Fredericks, H.D.B., Buckley, J., Baldwin, W.M., and Stremel-Campbell, K. (1983). The educational needs of the autistic adolescent. In E. Schopler and G.B. Mesibov (Eds.), *Autism in adolescents and adults* (pp. 79–109). New York: Plenum Press.

Heffner, E., and Balliett, E. (1976). *Utilization of existing community resources for delivery of mental health services to pre-school children.* Paper presented at 28th Annual Meeting of the American Association of Psychiatric Services for Children, San Francisco, November 1976.

Lansing, M.D., and Schopler, E. (1978). Individualized education: A public school model. In M. Rutter and E. Schopler (Eds.), *Autism: A reappraisal of concepts and treatment* (pp. 439–451). New York: Plenum Press.

Lovaas, O.I., Young, D.B., and Newsom, C.D. (1978). Childhood psychosis: Behavioral treatment. In B.B. Wolman, J. Egan, and A.O. Ross (Eds.), *Handbook of treatment of mental disorders in childhood and adolescence* (pp. 385–420). Englewood Cliffs, New Jersey: Prentice-Hall.

Mahler, M., in collaboration with Furer, M. (1968). *On human symbiosis and the vicissitudes of individuation. Vol. I, Infantile psychosis.* New York: International Universities Press.

Rutter, M. (1970). Autism: Educational issues. *Special Education*, *59*, 6–10.

Rutter, M. (1979). Autism: Psychopathological mechanisms and therapeutic approaches. In M. Bortner (Ed.), *Cognitive growth and development: Essays in memory of Herbert G. Birch* (pp. 273–298). New York: Brunner/Mazel.

Rutter, M., and Bartak, L. (1973). Special educational treatment of autistic children: A comparative study. II. Follow-up findings and implication for service. *Journal of Child Psychology and Psychiatry*, *14*, 241–270.

Rutter, M., and Sussenwein, F. (1971). A developmental and behavioral approach to the treatment of pre-school autistic children. *Journal of Autism and Childhood Schizophrenia*, *1*, 376–397.

Schopler, E. (1976). Toward reducing behavior problems in autistic children. In L. Wing (Ed.), *Early childhood autism* (pp. 221–245). Elmsford, New York: Pergamon Press.

Schopler, E., and Reichler, R.J. (1979). *Individualized assessment and treatment for autistic and developmentally disabled children. Vol. I, Psychoeducational Profile.* Baltimore: University Park Press.

Schopler, E., and Mesibov, G. (1985). *Communication problems in autism.* New York: Plenum Press.

Shapiro, T., and Sherman, M. (1984). Nursery schools. In T.B. Karasu (Ed.), *Psychiatric therapies: American Psychiatric Association Commission on Psychiatric Therapies* (pp. 630–636). Washington, DC: American Psychiatric Press.

Wing, J., and Wing, L. (1976). Provision of services. In L. Wing (Ed.), *Early childhood autism* (pp. 287–318). Elmsford, New York: Pergamon Press.

Wing, L. (1976). The principles of remedial education for autistic children. In L. Wing (Ed.), *Early childhood autism* (pp. 197–203). Elmsford, New York: Pergamon Press.

CHAPTER 8

FAMILY RESPONSE AND ADAPTATION TO A HANDICAP

Judith M. Levy

Children are born into families, and families must be considered whenever professionals address the problems of children. All too often professionals view parents and other family members as irksome and interfering without realizing the mutual impact of child and family. This mutual impact is true for handicapped children just as it is true for normal children. Adjustment to having a handicapped child is a slow and sometimes painful process. Helping professionals must work in concert with that process to help the child and his or her family.

FEELINGS EXPERIENCED BY PARENTS

Family members experience a gamut of emotions in response to having a handicapped child. Frequently, the emotions arise in a predictable progression from shock, to denial, to grief, to anger. Guilt is frequently present along the way. These emotions may occur in the order mentioned, or they may occur in a different order, sometimes overlapping, sometimes occurring simultaneously, or sometimes reversing temporarily. All of these responses are normal. Some of them are protective in that they permit a parent to function during the crisis immediately following diagnosis, when feelings of sadness and loss might hinder approprite functioning. However, some responses, although normal, impair a family's ability to adjust.

Shock

When a diagnosis is made, particularly if it is made at the child's birth, it may be so surprising, or so unanticipated, that the predominant experience of parents is generally one of shock and sometimes disorganization. People describe feeling as if they were falling apart and unable to cope, and needing someone to lean on. Particularly during conversations with professionals, parents may not hear what is said, and even very bright people may misunderstand because the turmoil inside them may prevent clear thinking.

If a diagnosis is made later, at some point after parents have had the opportunity to see their baby or live with their baby, the severity of the shock may be lessened. The more experience a family has had with their disabled child and the more severe (and obvious) the disability, the less shocking the diagnosis is likely to be. These parents have had time to see and experience for themselves the differences between their baby and a normal baby.

For children with less obvious disabilities, such as children with learning disabilities or attention deficit disorders, a diagnosis may not be made until the child is well into the school years. The parents, however, may have noticed since infancy that this child was different from their other children or different from the children of their friends. In fact, for some parents, the diagnosis is likely to come as a welcome relief in that it confirms their suspicions once and for all and may end a period of "shopping around" for someone to validate their own observations and perceptions. For these parents, a diagnosis means that they finally have an answer, which begins to chart a course for them.

People who are in shock require assistance to accomplish even the most basic tasks. Professionals must help these parents by providing concrete supports, such as assistance in making and keeping necessary appointments, arranging contacts with professionals such as school personnel and other consultants, and generally making specific recommendations based on their best professional judgment.

Denial

Denial of the problem, or the diagnosis, frequently is experienced by parents of handicapped children. The grim reality of the situation may be so difficult to accept, such an assault to the integrity of their egos, and so frightening to conceive of, that denial, even if it is only temporary, permits parents to avoid the hurt that the reality engenders. Just as it is difficult for parents to recognize that they have a handicapped child, so it may be difficult for professionals to impart this news to parents. Sometimes continuing denial by parents is subtly encouraged and reinforced by professionals who are uncomfortable telling them the truth when the news is not good. These professionals may, in fact, convince themselves that a particular child, given time, will grow out of his condition. Differences of opinion among professionals may also foster the continuance of parental denial by confirming for the parents that the diagnosis is uncertain.

Denial of the problem may manifest itself in many ways. Parents may miss appointments, refuse to follow through on professional advice, provide insufficient protection for the child in dangerous situations, expect more from the child than he or she is capable of, or move from doctor to doctor looking for another answer.

The key to helping a child when a parent appears to deny the problem is to detect if the parent provides the necessary services for the child. Most parents do proceed on the recommendations of professionals, despite their own disbelief and uncertainty. If, however, a parent refuses to follow professional advice, a decision must be made concerning the risk to the child. If necessary, appropriate protective steps must be taken to ensure the child's well-being. If, however, the parent's denial is not interfering with the child's progress, families must be respected for their decisions, provided with realistic feedback, and encouraged in their process of adjustment.

Sadness

Parents of handicapped children experience sadness because they did not have the child they anticipated having, and the child they do have will not fulfill their dreams. They are grieving for the child they expected, for themselves, and for the predicament in which they find themselves. They may also grieve for the child himself, who will never equal his peers in culturally acceptable measures, such as physical prowess, beauty, or self-sufficiency.

These parents frequently seem to be chronically sad or disappointed. On the surface they function well after the initial period of sadness and grief. They carry out their required roles as parents and partners. At certain times, however, particularly culturally important life events or rituals such as birthdays, graduation, weddings, or family gatherings, these parents experience a reawakening of the sadness. Olshansky (1962) termed this recurrent sadness "chronic sorrow," and Wikler, Wasow, and Hatfield (1980) noted that it persists for the parents into the adulthood of the handicapped child. At these times, the child's deviance from normal development is highlighted, causing the parents to face their loss again.

Parents experiencing initial or recurrent feelings of sadness may be helped by supportive counseling, which encourages expression of feelings in an accepting and normalizing atmosphere. Gradual exposure to other parents in similar circumstances is valuable to substantiate that others experience similar feelings and that it is possible to continue to cope despite feelings of profound sadness and loss. The slow but steady gains made by most handicapped children tend to mitigate a parent's grieving, as do the constant demands for care required by the child. Many parents say that circumstances dictate what a person is able to cope with and that generally there is little time for sadness or grief.

The father of a 12-year-old Jewish boy admitted to the Kennedy Institute in Baltimore for periodic reevaluation related that he and his wife have adjusted satisfactorily to their son's mental retardation, aggressive behavior, and placement in a residential school in another state. This year, however, normally the year for Bar Mitzvah, will be very difficult for them because their son will not attain this achievement. Although they have adapted and function normally on a daily basis, they know that this year they will be especially aware of their loss.

Anger

Parents of handicapped children have had their dreams frustrated, and the reality of life is sometimes very difficult for them and their children. It is natural to want to blame someone for this, and they do; frequently it is themselves, or professionals, or God. Parents who are angry are very difficult for professionals to work with. They complain that treatment services are insufficient, the hospital accommodations are second rate, or the school is not teaching their child anything. They appear to be very egocentric and not always concerned with the child's needs. It takes a patient and understanding professional to withstand the barrage of accusations that an angry parent can deliver. Unfortunately, parental attitudes can, at times, negatively affect the kind of treatment a child receives.

Parents whose overwhelming emotion is anger need the assistance of a skilled psychotherapist to help them understand the roots of the anger and how to cope with it. An angry person, however, rarely listens to professional advice. A social worker or other professional who develops a trusting relationship with the parent may broach this delicate subject. On the other hand, confrontation may be unnecessary so long as the anger is not interfering with the child's progress in any way. Caregivers and helping professionals working with children over the course of their development establish ongoing, supportive relationships with families, and may, in fact, observe the changing pattern of a parent's style of coping.

A 4-year-old boy ran into the street between two parked cars and was hit by an oncoming car. The mother, who was with her son, blamed herself for the accident. The boy suffered a closed head injury and was admitted to the Kennedy Institute, a center for treating handicapped children, for rehabilitation. The social worker attempted to speak directly with the mother about her expectations for the hospital stay and to provide support.

Although the mother did not refuse to speak with the social worker, her answers were curt and superficial, setting up a barrier that seemed impossible to penetrate. The only conversations the mother initiated from day to day were those concerning complaints about the nursing care, the food, and the fact that her son needed more therapy. The boy stayed in the hospital approximately 2 months. During that time, because the mother would not talk directly with the social worker or participate in the parents' group, the social worker took a different tack. She met the mother at her son's therapy, observing the treatment with her. She was also available in the corridor or the parents' lounge for informal chats about subjects seemingly irrelevant to the boy's condition. When the mother complained, the social worker listened and acted as an advocate when it was reasonable to do so. She did not argue with the mother. Finally, the mother began to stop by the social worker's office to say hello and report on her son's progress. By the end of her son's stay, this mother was able to share her anger as well as her fears with the social worker, and the anger began to dissipate. The social worker never put herself at odds with the mother by confronting her with her hostility and anger. Rather, she demonstrated acceptance of the mother's feelings, given the reality of her son's condition. Eventually the mother was able to look at the meaning of her behavior and move on to a more positive style of coping.

Guilt

A natural response to the occurrence of a misfortune is to look for the cause. Parents of handicapped children frequently look to themselves. In some few cases there is reason to feel guilty—for example, in situations involving alcohol or drug abuse, venereal disease, a family history of a particular condition, or child abuse or neglect. In most cases, however, the parents of handicapped children have no culpability whatever. This fact, though presented by professionals, nevertheless, does not stop parents from looking for reasons or blaming themselves. For some parents, religious convictions may reinforce this natural tendency by suggesting that this child's handicap is the punishment for a parent's transgressions. Societal attitudes founded in misinformation may add fuel to the fire. At its worst, guilt may cause one parent to project blame onto the other or onto the child. Anger directed toward the child only serves to increase the parents' sense of guilt. At this point, parents are rarely aware of the cause of their behavior, have little ability to support one another, and require professional assistance.

The first level of intervention in a situation involving guilt is medical counseling about the cause of the condition. This should be done as gently but frankly as possible and may require several sessions if the parents are not able to hear and accept the information clearly. Written documentation of the information is useful so that the parents can review the material as often as necessary. The involvement of a skilled mental health professional in the counseling is advisable so that any conflict between parents can be managed. If the information confirms a parent's responsibility for the disability, or if conflict between the parents persists, referral for individual or couples therapy by a social worker or other mental health professional should be strongly recommended. The suggestion for counseling can be made in a way that shows parents that their conflict is within the expected range of emotions under the circumstances. It should also openly identify the dysfunctional and destructive aspects of the conflict for the child as well as the parents.

Parents of handicapped children may feel guilty for reasons other than feeling responsible for the disability. Many parents, on seeing a handicapped child for the first time, secretly wish that the child would die or wonder, "Why is this happening to me?" Parents whose children have been in intensive care for weeks or months may begin to feel the personal strain as well as the toll on the whole family and wonder if it wouldn't be better for this child to die. Perhaps the parent considers the idea of placing the handicapped child out of the home. Regardless of what happens to the child, these parents carry the burden of knowing that they have had thoughts that they believe are inconceivable and unmentionable for a loving parent.

A parent burdened by this kind of guilt will benefit by attending a parent support group, at which it will become obvious that others have had similar feelings and thoughts. Sometimes parents react to their very negative thoughts by being either overprotective or underprotective of their children. Individual counseling as well as a parent support group will help these parents understand the roots of their behavior and encourage change.

SPECIAL ISSUES FOR FAMILIES WITH HANDICAPPED CHILDREN

The Parent–Child Relationship

Children are not just malleable organisms waiting to be shaped by an external socialization process. Each child has individual characteristics that not only affect the way the child is influenced by external forces but also help to shape the behavior of the socializers themselves (Bell and Harper, 1977). Optimal development will occur to the extent that the child's abilities, temperament, and motivational patterns occur in a consonant interaction with the demands and expectations of the environment (Chess, Fernandez, and Korn, 1980). Furthermore, it is assumed that the parent–child relationship will produce reciprocal satisfactions (Bentovim, 1972; Strickler, 1969). A state of symbiosis is necessary and normal for the development of both mother and child.

Unfortunately, disabled children may not have the resources to participate successfully in symbiotic relationships. Appearance, temperament, and physical and cognitive resources may affect parent–child interaction from the beginning. If a baby is visibly different from other babies, the parent is likely to respond in some unusual manner. The parent may experience uncertainty, discomfort, fear, horror, or sadness, and the feeling will be reflected in the interplay between parent and child.

A baby with Down syndrome, a cleft palate, spina bifida, or other physical anomaly not only may look different but also may require special handling and care, which adds to a parent's uncertainty and perhaps reluctance to hold and nurture the infant. A baby may be unusually cranky or irritable, a troublesome feeder, an inconsistent sleeper, or not cuddly or responsive. A baby with cerebral palsy who is very stiff and whose primitive reflexes are triggered easily may, in fact, appear to push a parent away when the baby postures involuntarily. Prior to obtaining professional counseling, a parent may interpret this behavior negatively and personally and will feel rejected and disappointed (Wetter, 1972).

Normally enjoyable and nurturing experiences, such as feeding, can be difficult if the baby has a poor suck, a tonic bite, or a swallowing abnormality. Even after diagnostic counseling, a mother who fails to feed her baby adequately and must seek professional advice may perceive that she has failed at the most basic of mothering functions. The feeding experience may thereafter be influenced by the mother's feelings of inadequacy as well as the baby's physical inadequacies. A vicious cycle may ensue if professional intervention is not obtained.

The baby's rate of development influences the parent–child relationship in that expected milestones are accomplished so slowly and so much later than normal that the parents do not feel reinforced for their efforts. The baby does not smile, laugh, or recognize the parents at the age that normal babies do, and its parents are left with only their own persistence and sense of responsibility to sustain them. Fathers in particular may feel lost unless they are involved from the beginning in professional counseling and training in the care of the baby. Otherwise, it is only the mother who begins to feel more at ease with the handicapped baby; the father becomes a peripheral and uninvolved figure.

For children whose disabilities are not visible or not diagnosed immediately, the symptoms may initially be interpreted behaviorally by both parents and professionals. Parents may respond negatively toward the child (Faerstein, 1981). These parents then have the additional burden of having to cope with the possibility that they contributed to the interactional problems and secondary emotional problems sometimes experienced by children with handicaps.

Samantha and her fraternal twin, Angela, were born when their parents were both in their late twenties and already had a normal, healthy 3-year-old daughter, Tracy. The mother's labor and delivery of the twins was very difficult, and Samantha was born with cerebral palsy, whereas Angela was not. The extent of Samantha's problems was not evident immediately, although both twins required extended hospitalization after birth. The mother, a registered nurse, attempted to breast feed both infants but was not able to get Samantha to suckle the breast or a bottle. Finally, the mother and Angela were discharged from the hospital, but Samantha was kept hospitalized because her feeding was so poor that professional intervention was required to devise a strategy to feed her orally. The family lived more than an hour's drive from the hospital, and with two young children at home, they were unable to visit more than once or twice a week. When visiting was possible, the mother generally came alone because the father was working or staying with the other girls. Visits were punctuated by a session with the occupational therapist, who taught the mother how to feed her baby.

Later on, this mother was able to describe how her own feelings of inadequacy with this baby influenced the bonding process. Feeling overwhelmed at home with the care of two children, and knowing that visits to Samantha in the hospital would only add to feelings of stress and inadequacy, it was easier to decide not to make the drive to the hospital. She convinced herself that other demands and outside factors prevented more frequent visits, when in fact, the bonding process had been affected by Samantha's feeding problems. The mother was not sufficiently attached to Samantha to motivate herself to overcome the very real obstacles which made it difficult for her to visit. Today, 3 years later, the mother and Samantha have a close, warm relationship, but one that continues to be affected by the characteristics of Samantha's cerebral palsy.

Loss

Parents of handicapped children can be expected to experience a sense of loss for the idealized child, the child that was fantasized about and expected (McCollum, 1984; Olshansky, 1962; Solnit and Stark,

1961). The loss of the awaited child must be dealt with before adjustment can be made to the child who is present, the handicapped child. Although a "real" death has not occurred, the process of beginning adjustment is similar to that postulated by Kubler-Ross (1969) after the actual death of a loved one. Parents and other family members, including siblings and grandparents, generally identify feelings that correspond to the stages of grieving that Kubler-Ross identifies. Although the loss of the idealized child is similar to the loss by death of a loved one, the difference is obvious. Parents of handicapped children do not have the time to grieve freely over the loss of the child they wished for because the child they have requires care and attention.

Parents whose children are disabled because of an accident or disease process must learn to cope with the loss of the child who actually existed prior to the accident but who now exists in an altered condition. For family members who have lived through long periods of uncertainty about the child's survival after the accident, the confirmation of his survival with a disability assumes different meaning. These parents may have been better prepared for death than for life with disability. For them, anger and denial may be the most prolonged and intense of the feelings during the grieving process. Ambivalence is heightened as parents relive the events leading up to the accident that left them with a handicapped child. In addition to their own adjustment, parents of children with sufficient cognitive capacity will have to help the children themselves deal with the loss of their physical and mental capacities. Questions of physical appearance, academic competence, and acceptance by peers will be uppermost in these youngsters' concerns. Ambivalence of their own concerning whether it was better to live or die may arise to mirror that of their parents.

These children and their families can be helped by counseling, which assures them that their response is normal, and by involvement with groups of people adjusting to similar circumstances. For families who have more dysfunctional and perhaps self-destructive reactions, individual psychotherapy is warranted.

Values

The characteristics of the ideal child are determined by the culture as well as by individual preferences. The ideal child represents the values of the parent that are incorporated from society at large and the parents' own family. American culture values independence, academic achievement, good looks, and at least average athletic ability. Parents whose children are disabled know that they will never achieve in at least one, and perhaps in all, of these areas. They are, thus, faced with the dilemma of how to view this child and where to fit him or her into their value system.

A primary role of parenting is the transmission of culture through children. Parents know that their children must assume a culturally valued role in our society to be viewed as successful (Levine, 1980). If a society rejects a child, the child is prevented from assuming a valued role, and the parent is prevented from carrying out his or her responsibility; as a result, the children as well as their parents are devalued. These parents raise their children in a "social void" (Roskies, 1972). The development of sheltered workshops and other protected employment for handicapped people who are unable to be employed competitively permits the attainment of a culturally valued role. Parents of children who are more severely handicapped do not have this option. Handicapped people who are cognitively normal or nearly normal are acutely aware of the need to fulfill a culturally valued role and strive to do so.

Parents must find a place for their handicapped child in their value system so that he or she fits into their frame of reference in a positive way (Wolfensberger, 1967). This frame of reference may be religious or secular. A parent who is religious may interpret a handicapped child as a "gift from God" because the parent is viewed by God as being capable of providing the specialized care required by the child. A secular interpretation may be that helping a handicapped child reach his or her maximum potential is one of life's challenges that both parents accept and share.

Stigma

Persons who deviate from the norm are stigmatized. Goffman (1963) noted that a stigmatized person is one who "is reduced in our minds from a whole and usual person to a tainted and discounted one." The role society expects of handicapped people is characterized by incompetence, helplessness, and deviance (Fewell and Gelb, 1983). Therefore, stigma may preclude other, more normal roles even when an individual's disability would not.

The issue of the handicapped child's difference is faced by all family members. For parents, the stigma is initially felt as an assault to their own egos because they have internalized cultural values. Thus, the management of their child's difference may become an all-encompassing preoccupation for them. Finding a niche for the child in their value system is the parents' first step toward coping successfully with the difference within the family. The parents' acceptance of their own handicapped child strengthens their presentation to the community.

People who are different stand out immediately. Today, with increasing numbers of disabled people in the community, difference is becoming more acceptable. It does not go unnoticed, however. A parent shopping with an obviously handicapped youngster is bound to be the subject of stares if not actual questioning about the diagnosis and cause of the disability. The intrusion may be rude or reflective of genuine concern. At its worst, it may be pity. In any case, it is the rare parent who can respond to such questioning with equanimity. Moreover, stigma can erect barriers between friends who, although anxious to help, have insufficient or incorrect information and may refrain from contacts because of what they perceive to be an intrusion. The same is true for grandparents and other family members, who may be uncertain about how to help the child and his family.

For some handicapped children, the issue of stigma relates less to physical appearance than it does to behavior. For parents of children who appear normal but who act differently, the immediate problems are those of responsibility and control. In United States society, parents are responsible for their children and must control their behavior. Learning disabled children who do not achieve in school or autistic or hyperactive children whose behavior is out of control do not necessarily look different from other children. But the social and psychological consequences may be even more negative when the condition is not visible (Stein and Jessup, 1982).

In addition, brothers and sisters of handicapped children experience stigma as a backdrop to their lives. By association they are different and stigmatized too. This is particularly a problem if the handicapped child attends the same school as his or her sibling(s). Even the well-adjusted sibling can experience serious problems coping with the issues of difference during adolescence. Teenagers must break away from the family to establish their own separate identity. This is easiest to do if the family is a "normal" family that is accepted in the community and has, therefore, projected a sense of pride and stability, which has been incorporated by the teenager. If, however, the teenager recognizes that because of a handicapped child, the family has a marginal status, then so does he or she, and his or her own identity is marred. Additionally, in the course of the normal rejection of the family that occurs during adolescence, this teenager may feel ambivalence and guilt because society at large has already rejected his or her family. Stigma may, in a paradoxical way, interfere with the primary task of the adolescent.

Concerns for the Future

Parents are always concerned about the future of their children. For most parents, however, the vicissitudes of raising children are mediated by the near certainty that most children do manage to grow up and leave home to begin a life of their own. Parents of handicapped children are less certain of this because, depending on the nature and severity of the disability, their child may never be able to live alone or without care.

For parents of the most severely disabled children, the situation may be easier to deal with because it is clear that their child will always need care. The problem then becomes one of finding the necessary care for an adult child. The tide has changed in American culture, however. It is no longer easy to place a person in an institution because of a mental or physical disability. Nor would many families wish to. Nevertheless, the burden of caring for severely handicapped children can take its toll on families. By the time the child has reached adulthood, these families require assistance in continuing to provide total care for their children. If there are other children in the family, they may have contributed significantly to the provision of care. Now these children are grown and are moving out at a time when the physical capabilities of the parents are on the decline. For children handicapped to a lesser degree and able to carry out more of their own self-care, supervised group home living may be a possibility, with the major deterrent being the insufficient number of these facilities.

For parents of children who are diagnosed as being learning disabled or having attention-deficit hyperactivity disorder, the future is in some ways more difficult because it is such a mystery. What will they be able to accomplish? What strategies will they learn to compensate for their deficits? Will they find a trade or occupation that lends itself to their strengths and minimizes their shortcomings? With appropriate education and strong parental support, these children will probably find such a trade. Yet parents still must learn to live with the uncertainty of these conditions, which results from the amorphous and as yet little understood nature of the disabilities themselves (Willner and Crane, 1979).

In the United States, because most handicapped people over 18 years are eligible for Supplemental Security Income and Medical Assistance through the Social Security system, the strain of financial security is not so severe for parents. As this is not enough to support an adult under normal circumstances, however, special arrangements must be made if the handicapped person is not living with a family member.

Siblings are concerned about their future responsibility for their handicapped brother or sister, especially after the parents have died. Specifically they have questions about long-term care and the quality of life (Powell and Ogle, 1985). Assuming that basic necessities such as shelter, food and clothing are provided for, what provisions can be made for the day-to-day "work" of handicapped adults? Most parents and siblings want their handicapped family member to be occupied in a way that has value in our culture. Competitive employment is therefore the most desirable. For those unable to manage the competitive world, sheltered employment is sought by many people. For persons unable to perform work in the traditional sense because of physical or mental disabilities, some educational pursuit is seen as the next best approach. This may take many forms, depending on the person's capabilities. For some persons, this may involve arts and crafts and socializing activities at a day program; for others, who are more capable mentally, it is all the more important to develop stimulating programs to provide them with a raison d'être and to forestall depression, anger, and bitterness.

DAY-TO-DAY REALITIES OF RAISING A HANDICAPPED CHILD

To begin with, parents of normal children can rely on a variety of available resources for consultation about child rearing. Parents of handicapped children do not have the same resources. Usually, they cannot refer to their own personal development, observations of other children, other parent–child interaction, or informal conversation with friends, neighbors, and grandparents. Especially at first, these parents want to discuss all decisions with someone whom they trust because they do not have sufficient information to make reasoned decisions for themselves. Consider Samantha, mentioned previously, who had severe feeding problems. At first, when Samantha went home, her mother made long-distance phone calls to the occupational therapist for consultation if a feeding problem arose. Gradually, she began to feel confident enough in her own knowledge to make certain modifications and decisions on her own.

Similarly, it is difficult for many parents of handicapped children to find a babysitter. This not only prevents them from meeting their own needs for relaxation, but it may also interfere with the parenting of other children in the family. Normally families use grandparents, other family members, or paid babysitters when it is necessary for them to leave the home. If parents are at a loss as to how to care for their own handicapped youngsters, however, it is understandable that others would be too.

In addition, parents of handicapped children experience stigmatized social interactions daily. They face financial strain because their medical insurance does not cover all of the treatment and services that the child requires. They may even have no medical insurance at all. Equipment necessary to care for the handicapped child may break down and need repairs. The burden of care for a severely disabled youngster needing total care is endless and frequently requires the assistance of all family members. Fathers and teenaged brothers can lift or transport up and down stairs, but they should not be called on to bathe a teenaged severely handicapped girl. Younger siblings are frequently called on to carry out tasks such as household chores earlier than normal because of their handicapped sibling.

The following quotation sums up the daily reality of parenting a handicapped child:

> There are some similarities in the experience of all parents of children with exceptional needs. They encounter the dilemmas of finding appropriate services, of marshalling resources, of explaining their child's needs as well as their own needs to a society that tells them in subtle ways that their child is unworthy. Parents enumerate common experiences with service professionals as well: They tell of being forced to interact continually with professionals who do not seem to realize how it feels to be a parent or who view parents as unable to understand what the problems are and yet, nevertheless, expect parents to be understanding and cooperative, passive and appreciative (Fewell and Gelb, 1983).

THE FAMILY LIFE CYCLE

This section examines the impact of a handicapped child on the family life cycle. The concept of the family life cycle reflects the "reciprocal influence between individual growth processes and family coping patterns and forces one to look at the family as the most potent milieu in which growth and change occur" (Rhodes, 1977). According to Erikson (1963), the tasks and needs facing persons at a particular time can be understood in terms of an interactive process through which people seek to balance their own drive toward self-actualization with society's expectations. Rhodes (1977) suggests that in families there are average expectable milestones, characterized by phase-specific tasks and needs. A life cycle approach to understanding families juxtaposes interdependent life tasks of individual family members with developmental family tasks. Tasks of a given life stage are accomplished by utilizing opportunities and resources. When there is a deficit in opportunities or resources, tasks cannot be accomplished (O'Hara and Levy, 1984).

For the purpose of this chapter, the conceptualizations of Erikson (1963) and Rhodes (1977) will be used as reference for the stages of individual and family life cycles respectively. Tables 8–1 through 8–6 are adapted from O'Hara and Levy (1984). They represent the needs and tasks of persons as well as the family as a whole, in interaction with

TABLE 8-1.
Life Stage A: Establishing the Family
Life Cycle Needs, Tasks, and Problems of Families with Handicapped Children
in the Prenatal Period

Family	Parents
Tasks	*Tasks*
Intimacy versus idealization or disillusionment	Intimacy versus isolation
Needs	*Needs*
Establish consensus of values and roles	Separation from family of origin
Plan pregnancy and prenatal care	Incorporation of spousal role into identity
Problems	*Problems*
High-risk pregnancy	Drug or alcohol abuse
Poor prenatal care	Physical spouse abuse
Adolescent parent	Exposure to environmental toxins
	Family history of handicapping condition

Adapted from Erikson (1963) and Rhodes (1977).

one another throughout the life cycle. The tables identify needs and problems specific to handicapped children and their families. The tables cover the prenatal period through 21 years of age. The remaining portion of this chapter focuses on critical junctures in the life cycle of families: the childbearing years, the preschool and school years, the teenage years, and the young adult years.

Effect on the Normal Family Life Cycle of the Birth of a Handicapped Child

According to Erikson, the task of the parents in *life stage B, the childbearing years*, is generativity versus stagnation. Generativity refers to the mutual teaching-learning process between generations that satisfies the parents' need to be needed and the children's need to be guided to productivity in the particular culture (see Table 8-2).

When a handicapped baby is born to a couple, the couple usually has had no preparation for a baby whose special needs require extraordinary care. A handicapped baby puts the parents in a quandary about whether or not they will be able to raise this baby to a productive station both because of the baby's limitations and because of their own lack of competence. This then affects the development of their identity as parents and makes it difficult for them to establish a sense of

TABLE 8-2.
Life Stage B: The Childbearing Years
Life Cycle Needs, Tasks, and Problems of Families with Handicapped Children
from Birth to 18 Months

Child	Family	Parents
Tasks	*Tasks*	*Tasks*
Basic trust versus mistrust	Replenishment versus turning inward	Generativity versus stagnation
Needs	*Needs*	*Needs*
Effective parenting	Possible modifications	Establishment of
Early diagnosis and treatment	in values and roles to accommodate handicapped child	parental identity
Problems	*Problems*	*Problems*
Irregular feeding and sleeping patterns	Adjustment of roles and responsibilities	Self-doubt in parenting role
Slow development of gross and fine motor skills	Failure to establish mutuality in parent–child interaction	Decisions about future children
Temperamental and behavioral problems	Value disorientation	Emotional inability to parent a "difficult" child
Lack of diagnosis	Reactions of siblings, extended family, and friends	Inability to provide adequate care
	Beginning involvement of professionals in family life	

Adapted from O'Hara and Levy (1984).

mutuality with their child. Because of the difference between this child and the one they expected, the parents do not know how to proceed and may experience grief at the loss of the idealized child, as was described previously.

A couple in life stage B should have established consensus on values and role organization within the family during the previous stage (see Table 8–1, *life stage A: establishing the family.*) The birth of a child who is different may call into question the values agreed on as vital to the continued viability of the family. The ideal solution for this problem is for the couple to work through the question of values with an understanding of the social and cultural contributions to their attitudes so that they can fit this child into the value system of their family. Problems arise frequently because the parents are psychologically unavailable to each other owing to their individual grief and mourning processes. Couples who have achieved real intimacy prior to this

TABLE 8-3.
Life Stage C: The Toddler Years
Life Cycle Needs, Tasks, and Problems of Families with Handicapped Children aged 18 Months to 3 Years

Child	Family	Parents
Tasks	*Tasks*	*Tasks*
Autonomy versus shame and doubt	Replenishment versus turning inward	Generativity versus stagnation
Needs	*Needs*	*Needs*
Effective parenting	Incorporation of difference into family values	Ongoing development of parents
Early socialization and play		Maintenance of community ties
Early diagnosis and treatment	Attention to sibling needs	
Problems	*Problems*	*Problems*
Delayed development prevents autonomy	Disproportionate emotional resources used for "difficult" child	Inability to meet needs of spouse or of other children
Beginning of self-doubt	Shift in focus of family life	Sense of inadequacy
	Increasing frustration with slow development	Physical burden of care
	Coping with stigma	

Adapted from O'Hara and Levy (1984).

crisis will be able to help each other through the grieving process, the redefinition of their values, and the restructuring of roles within the family that may be necessary. These couples will respond to the gentle but focused guidance of astute clinicians who are able to observe where the process of adjustment is stuck.

The task for the family in life stage B (and also in life stages C and D, Tables 8–3 and 8–4) is emotional replenishment. The nurturers must be replenished so they can continue to nurture the child as well as each other and other family members. The alternative to replenishment is turning inward, individual self-absorption. A baby who has special and unusual needs quickly drains the provider of physical and emotional resources. If the parents do not recognize the need or are temporarily unable to provide support to one another, support must be mobilized from other sources. Friends and other extended family members may be able to meet the needs of the parents by providing supportive

TABLE 8-4.
Life Stage D: The Preschool and School Years
Life Cycle Needs, Tasks, and Problems of Families with Handicapped Children
aged 3 to 12 Years

Child	Family	Parents
Tasks	*Tasks*	*Tasks*
Initiative versus guilt	Replenishment versus	Generativity versus
Industry versus	turning inward	stagnation
inferiority	Individuation of family	
	members	
Needs	*Needs*	*Needs*
Management of	Consensus on values	Marital stability
differentness	and roles	Career opportunity (for
Initial diagnosis for	Acceptance of child	some)
some disabilities	and family limitations	
Ongoing medical care	Normal expectations	
Peer relationships	for siblings	
Correct educational		
planning		
Achievement of sexual		
identity		
Problems	*Problems*	*Problems*
Social isolation	Inadequate financial	Lost career and
Inadequate learning	resources	developmental
resources	Family breakdown	opportunities
Lack of definitive	Pressure for siblings to	Ongoing isolation
diagnosis	achieve or to fill	
Parental over- and	inappropriate roles	
underprotection	within family	
	Lack of family support	
	services	

Adapted from O'Hara and Levy (1984).

conversations or substitute care on a temporary basis. Unfortunately, older children may be called on inappropriately to fill this role, and this may set into motion a premature process of development for the sibling, which prevents the accomplishment of his or her own appropriate life cycle needs and tasks.

Jeremy was born to a middle income, intelligent couple in their twenties. They had been married 6 years, had a 4-year-old son, Brad, owned a house, and planned to have two children. The mother stayed home with the children in a development of single family homes about a 45 minutes' drive from the University Hospital where Jeremy was born. The couple described a good,

TABLE 8–5.
Life Stage E: The Teenage Years
Life Cycle Needs, Tasks, and Problems of Families with Handicapped Children
aged 13 to 18 Years

Adolescent	Family	Parents
Tasks	*Tasks*	*Tasks*
Identity versus role confusion	Companionship versus isolation	Generativity versus stagnation
Needs	*Needs*	*Needs*
Achieve healthy sexual identity	Negotiation of new parent–child relationship and roles	Preparation for eventual separation of children
Acquire skills for maximum independence		
Correct educational placement		
Vocational planning		
Consideration of capacity for independent living		
Peer relationships		
Human sexuality training		
Recreation		
Problems	*Problems*	*Problems*
Social isolation	Rejection of handicapped teen by adolescent siblings	Allowing independence
Incorrect school placement	Lack of community support to plan for adulthood	
Lack of appropriate vocational resources		
Inability to live independently		
Overprotection by parents		
Pregnancy		

Adapted from O'Hara and Levy (1984).

mutually supportive relationship but very little contact with extended family members on either side. This couple felt very strongly that they had only themselves to rely on. At birth, Jeremy did not do well, and a heart problem was detected. His feeding was difficult and he would not nurse. He went home with his family after several weeks in the hospital, taking formula. A follow-up visit was scheduled with the cardiologist. Jeremy's parents became

TABLE 8–6.
Life Stage F: Family As A Launching Center
Life Cycle Needs, Tasks, and Problems of Families with Handicapped Children
aged 18 to 21 Years

Young Adult	Family	Parents
Tasks	*Tasks*	*Tasks*
Intimacy versus isolation	Regrouping versus binding or expulsion	Generativity versus stagnation
		Ego integrity versus despair
Needs	*Needs*	*Needs*
Preparation for independence	Negotiation of roles of adult children	Renewal of marital relationship
Self-fulfillment in adult roles	Care of family member who cannot achieve full independence	
Adult legal rights versus establishment of guardianship		
Socialization and heterosexual relationships		
Planning for adult living		
Problems	*Problems*	*Problems*
Lack of opportunity for employment or independent living	Family inability to allow independence	Inability to move on from parental role
Failure to achieve adulthood	Lack of community resources to support move from family	
Criminal exploitation		

Adapted from O'Hara and Levy (1984).

concerned because he was not progressing normally. Their pediatrician said that because of the problems at birth and the heart problem, it was expected that he would lag a little initially. Finally, at 1 year, Jeremy was still not eating well, gaining weight, or sitting up. The parents had experienced a year of sleepless nights, uncertainty, and anguish. They decided to ask their pediatrician to recommend a specialist who might be able to give them answers about Jeremy. The pediatrician recommended a hospital that specialized in the diagnosis, evaluation, and treatment of developmentally disabled children.

During the evaluation period, the social worker spoke with both parents and learned that although their relationship was basically solid, their efforts to cope with Jeremy's deficits took quite different paths. The father, who participated less in Jeremy's care, was able to intellectualize about the slowness of his milestones by pointing to the birth history and physical problems. He did not want to discuss his fears and anxieties about Jeremy's condition, even with his wife. The mother, now raising her second child, was acutely aware that something was wrong, could not deny it to herself, and needed to be able to verbalize her fears. She confided to the social worker that the marital relationship was under great strain. They were not able to share their thoughts with each other, and they had not gone out without the children since Jeremy's birth because they were afraid to leave him with anyone. With the exception of the paternal grandmother, most of their extended family was unaware of Jeremy's status since birth. Although their friends were sympathetic, this couple really did not share their worst fears with anyone and would not ask their friends for moral support or even babysitting help.

Jeremy was diagnosed as having a rare, genetically transmitted syndrome that involved cardiac deficits, mental retardation, and metabolic problems. The counseling with the parents involved a developmental pediatrician and the social worker. In addition to providing accurate diagnostic information, they talked with this couple about normal parental reactions to having a handicapped child, reassuring them that what they were experiencing was to be expected. The difference in parental coping styles was brought into the open so they could begin to understand what prevented them from supporting one another. This couple was advised to begin to take time to listen to one another, to identify the value dilemma they were facing, and to begin to ask for some support from friends or family by sharing information with them. The therapists instructed the parents in feeding techniques and how to encourage Jeremy in his next physical milestone, sitting up.

The father was in the process of changing jobs, which meant that he would change insurance coverage and that the family would move to a different county, much farther from the metropolitan area. The social worker helped the father look into insurance coverage for Jeremy under the new policy and investigated the provisions for handicapped children in the new school system. Jeremy continued to come to the hospital for routine follow-up. The parents were pleased with the school system, Jeremy's progress, and their new home. They were beginning to understand and to share their thoughts and feelings with each other, although they continued to be somewhat isolated from outside contacts with family or friends.

The Family with a Handicapped Child of School Age

The tasks for children in *life stage D (the preschool and school years)* who have attained a sense of self or autonomy in *life stage C (toddlers)* are the development first of initiative and then of industry (see Tables 8–4 and 8–3, respectively). First, these 3- to 12-year-old children must plan, and undertake activities for the sake of being active and on the move. Second, they must learn to win recognition by producing things, by using the tools of the culture (Erikson, 1963). In families whose children are of school age, individual children are becoming increasingly independent, and concerns shift from family to individual agendas. The major task of this stage is for the children to begin to develop an identity that is not rooted entirely in roles within the family. The danger is that a family may preserve interpersonal harmony at the expense of individual difference.

Parents continue to need to replenish themselves so that they are able to nurture each other as well as their children. The burden of caring for a child with special needs means that replenishment is even more important, but it is, ironically, even harder to achieve: Babysitters for handicapped children are scarce and expensive. The needs of the handicapped child may be so time consuming that there is no time during the day for parents to meet their own replenishment needs. The other children in the family demand "equal time," and most parents will attend to their children before themselves.

Parents and other children in the family must continue to make adaptations in role organization and value orientations. The special needs of the school-aged handicapped child may force all family members, including siblings, to contribute in unanticipated ways to his or her care and general family maintenance. Brothers and sisters may be called on to perform household chores normally carried out by parents so that parents are able to perform therapeutic tasks for the handicapped youngster or take the child for medical appointments. One or both parents may be required to work longer hours or have two jobs to meet the additional financial demands of caring for the handicapped child. What is more likely, however, is that one parent will have to forego career goals or a job because care for the handicapped child is unavailable. If both parents do work, however, brothers or sisters may be the after-school babysitters, thereby causing them to curtail their extracurricular activities with peers. Siblings may have to learn to adapt to insufficient parental attention for themselves. This may occur because the parent is caring for the handicapped child or because the parent has not worked through feelings of denial or guilt and thus spends excessive time with the handicapped child.

The incorporation of difference into the family's value system and the management of stigma are two crucial tasks facing families during the preschool and school years. The handicapped child is growing, his or her differences are probably more obvious, either physically or behaviorally, and he or she is more often in the public eye. The child begins to attend school. Depending on the nature and severity of the handicap, he or she may attend a special school or the neighborhood school. A special school bus may pick the child up in the neighborhood, making the difference obvious to everyone. If the child attends the neighborhood school, a sibling may be required to walk him or her to school, and the sibling will have to bridge the gap between the family and peers. Although some close friends may have visited the family home and expressed acceptance of the handicapped child, the jump to public exposure on a large scale will be inescapable and may prove difficult. A brother or sister may have had the choice about joining the handicapped child on other public excursions but not about joining him or her in attending school.

Parents whose children are of school age are most likely to be involved with their own task of generativity versus stagnation. The generativity of parents—that is, their need to teach and guide their children—will be satisfied by the ongoing needs of the handicapped child as well as those of their other children. The handicapped child's developmental differences are, in this stage, becoming all too obvious, however, and the parents will begin to wonder if their efforts will ever lead to maturity or if they and the child will be ''frozen'' at this point forever. In reality the child's delays and abnormalities are just that— frozen. This child may not be walking, talking, or toilet trained. The child may have to be dressed and bathed. If the child's disabilities are at the less severe end of the spectrum, the parents and other family members may have held out hope for a fairly normal future. Introduction to the academic world will either substantiate or repudiate that dream.

The entire family must come to grips with the difference between their family and others in a way that permits the maintenance of self-esteem and the growth of family members. This involves the recognition of strengths as well as limitations. Family members must reassess goals and appreciate small gains and victories.

Tracy is a 6-year-old girl diagnosed as having severe mental retardation and cerebral palsy, as well as a seizure disorder, which is only partially controlled by medication. Her brother Bobby is 9, and her sister Suzanne is 13. Tracy's father has a good job in state government and is completing studies for a graduate degree in night school. Tracy's mother is a licensed practical nurse but currently stays at home with the children. They live in a development of single family homes about a 30 minute drive from the metropolitan area, where many families move because housing is more affordable and because it is considered a more wholesome place to raise children. The parents have a relationship based on understanding and mutual support. They have passed on this caring attitude to their children.

Tracy was a normal child until the age of 2 years when she picked up a tack from the floor and swallowed it. It lodged in her trachea, causing her to stop breathing, and she suffered anoxic brain damage. Her brother Bobby reportedly is responsible for the tack's being on the floor, although he has never been "blamed" by his parents. As Tracy recovered, it became clear to the medical staff that she was now a severely handicapped little girl. Besides the seizure disorder, her major problem was feeding, and a gastrostomy tube was inserted, which permitted the provision of nutrients by tube directly into her stomach. This, plus another procedure, reduced the likelihood that she would aspirate food into her lungs and allowed her to grow. When Tracy went home from the hospital, her parents kept her in their room at night and hardly slept for fear that she would die. The parents, who grieved the loss of their child as she had been, managed to comfort each other as well as their two other children.

It is a tribute to the strength of the parents' relationship that this family has nurtured its members sufficiently to prevent the turning inward or self-absorption of the individual members. Despite the parents' refusal to use the services of a sitter or trained respite care provider for 4 years, the siblings continued to participate in school and extracurricular activities, and the parents seemed to find quiet moments for each other. A maternal aunt was called in about once a year to stay with the children while the parents went to a function that they considered important. The family's religious faith was a major source of replenishment. All family members, including Suzanne and Bobby, take pleasure in Tracy's small victories. Because Tracy is very seriously handicapped, she attends a different school from her sister and brother. The neighborhood, including peers of Bobby and Suzanne, accepts Tracy. The pressure of stigma from other children in Bobby's and Suzanne's school environment is lessened because Tracy attends a different school and because the parents have fostered such a "normal" existence for their children. Tracy is not hidden, and the other children are not deprived of important developmental experiences. Bobby and Suzanne engage in the normal sibling rivalry, but do share the ability to confide in one another.

Although certain roles and responsibilities are linked to specific family members, there is a sharing of responsibilities by the parents, which demonstrates caring and cooperation to the other children. Probably because their own needs are satisfied sufficiently, these children are willing to help out in the care of Tracy and their home. Despite continued progress, this family knows that Tracy will always be severely handicapped. Tracy has not achieved a sense of self or autonomy, expected in life stage C (toddlers), let alone the initiative and industry of life stage D, because she is severely retarded as well as physically disabled. It is beginning to dawn on the family that Tracy's limited potential has the power to ''arrest'' individual and family life cycles.

This family demonstrates generally positive adjustment to the handicapping condition of one of its children. The fact that the disability resulted from a traumatic injury after birth adds a special dimension in that the family is faced with the loss of Tracy as she was, while she is still with them. The danger for this family is the overextension of parenting to maintain for the children a so-called normal family life to the exclusion of nourishment for the parents themselves. The energy expended on parenting has to take its toll on this couple.

Additionally, Bobby has some understandable sensitivity to the circumstances surrounding Tracy's accident. The manifestation of this is an aura of seriousness and intensity, which is relieved by talking about his sister's life and accomplishments and expressing his concerns for his parents. In the future, individual counseling may be beneficial in helping him adjust to Tracy's condition. Both parents and children attended a workshop for families that addressed the concerns of parents and siblings separately. They have also contributed their time by participating in panel discussions for the education of professional audiences.

The Family with a Handicapped Adolescent or Young Adult

The task for children at *life stage E, the teenage years,* is the development of a singular identity that feels comfortable and acceptable to them in their particular culture (see Table 8–5). Parents continue to provide guidance to their children with the goal of productive adulthood. The task for the family is to shift their energies from family concerns to individual interests. The struggle for parents is to prepare for an identity that is not defined by their roles and responsibilities within the family. Parents and children must begin to develop companionship both within and outside the family circle. This is the precursor of the major shifts in family relationships that occur in *life stage F, family as a launching center* (see Table 8–6). Normal siblings, with increasing self-sufficiency, should be propelled into the larger community. The task for them is the establishment of their own identities.

What of the family that has not been able to nourish its members sufficiently or is unable to tolerate difference? This family may tighten its boundaries around offspring, thereby preventing them from moving outside. These families believe that the only way to survive is by continuing their attachment to one another in a pseudomutual organization—that is, one that is outwardly satisfying to its members but that does not recognize the autonomy or singularity of individual members. A family with a severely handicapped child, whose inner resources have been depleted and whose experience with environmental resources has been less than satisfactory, may hold on to its members in an effort to protect them. This, then, prolongs the parenting role and arrests the life cycle.

Siblings who are encouraged to venture outside of family boundaries have significant pressures to deal with. The normal sibling may very well be concerned about his or her own potential to produce a deficient offspring, the ability to find a mate, and his or her responsibility for the handicapped brother or sister in the future. At this stage, brothers or sisters who previously made a good adjustment to the handicapped child may surprise everyone by rejecting him or her. The rejection may be manifested by refusal to participate in care, having little patience, or unwillingness to be seen in public with the handicapped child. The peer pressure to conform is so great that the management of difference may be impossible.

Both the handicapped adolescent and the parents are coping with biological, psychological, and social issues that they may not understand. For parents of learning disabled teenagers, a major problem may be their inability to discontinue their protective role. Vocational counseling, maximum independence, and peer relationships are major needs of the learning disabled adolescent and young adult.

A more severely disabled teenager presents different issues. Sexuality may be the primary concern for parents. If the teenager is in the mild to moderate range of the spectrum, this child will most likely identify with other teenagers but not have the ability to understand the forces affecting him or to make sound judgments. Most parents worry about the sexual vulnerability of boys as well as girls—ambulatory as well as nonambulatory teenagers. Female adolescents also have menses to contend with. If they cannot manage on their own, the parents must do it for them.

In *life stage F (the family as a launching center)*, parents must prepare for the eventual separation from their children. How can a parent separate from a child who will never achieve independence? What guarantees do they have that these children will be taken care of after their deaths? Parents have difficulty developing an identity that is not defined by parenting roles because they must continue to parent for an indefinite period of time. In addition, at this point, the perception of normal siblings that they are expected to care for their handicapped brother or sister may be accurate.

Gwen is a twin whose cerebral palsy and mild mental retardation were interpreted by her parents as a life challenge for them. Gwen's older brother, John, as well as her twin sister Anne, are straight A students in school. Both siblings have adjusted well to having a handicapped sister. In previous years they worked at a camp for handicapped children during the summer. The parents both work and manage a very hectic schedule. All of the children's needs are addressed, and the family generally manages a special weekend away once a month. The parents provide good support to one another, but they are having difficulty incorporating the behavior of all three children into their frame of reference. In line with their own identification of Gwen as a "challenge," they expect that everyone will work to his or her potential, and no complaining is permitted. The family's physical and emotional resources are becoming depleted, however.

For the past 12 years, John, now 16 years old, has demonstrated increasing anger and hostility toward Gwen by teasing her until she cries and refusing to help her when either she or their parents make a request. Anne has a rather patronizing attitude toward Gwen and was heard speaking very harshly to her following Gwen's surgery when Gwen sounded as if she was "whining." To the parents' credit is the fact that they have encouraged both John and Anne to participate in their own activities and to choose their own summer jobs.

Until very recently, the parents have not permitted Gwen to use a wheelchair in the house, expecting her to crawl or use a walker. Because of the slowness of these methods, Gwen's increasing size, and the necessity for as much independence as possible, however, the parents are having to reconsider their expectations. Despite their acceptance of the "challenge," their goals may be unattainable for Gwen. The future for Gwen is in question as the parents consider how they expect to spend their lives after their other two children become independent. The future is not so simple for Gwen, but these parents are ready for the next family life stage, in which their roles are not defined solely by parenting.

Shanika is a 16-year-old girl diagnosed as being mildly mentally retarded. Both parents were reared in an institution for the mentally deficient. Shanika's 18-year-old brother reportedly is retarded as well and dropped out of school before graduation. Both sister and brother have been raised since infancy by a maternal aunt who is employed and is buying her own home. A maternal uncle and grandfather live in the home but do not work. The aunt brought Shanika for counseling because of behavior problems at home and at school. Shanika had been mainstreamed for 2 years previously and was failing in a ninth grade classroom for the second time. She was truant, did not do her homework, and stayed out at night into the morning hours. Shanika had a boyfriend and had had one abortion at age 15. She had birth control pills, which she took inconsistently.

Her aunt feared that Shanika would become pregnant again or get involved with drugs. Her aunt correctly perceived that Shanika was very much influenced by peer pressure and could be persuaded to do almost anything. The aunt was exhausted and expected that at 16 years Shanika should begin to act more "grown up" and use "common sense." She talked and lectured constantly in an effort to teach Shanika what was "right." But Shanika wanted to do what her friends were doing. Her friends were permitted to stay out late, and Shanika wanted to do the same. Although she did not want to have a baby, she thought that the birth control pill caused water retention, so she did not want to use that method of birth control. The aunt and the clinic justifiably contended that, for Shanika, it was the most reliable method with the least risk to her.

Shanika and her aunt expressed mutual love and support, as Shanika experienced the normal struggles of adolescence. The exacerbating factors, however, were the inappropriate school placement and the unrealistic expectations of the aunt for Shanika's behavior. The school placement put Shanika in daily contact with peers chronologically the same age, but socially and intellectually more advanced. Her biological drives were similar, as was her need to belong, but her capacity to understand the biological impact of adolescent hormones and to make sound judgments was seriously deficient. She was in a situation that she was poorly equipped to handle.

The aunt knew that Shanika was retarded and functioned at a mental age much younger than her chronological age. After 18 years of raising her sister's two children, however, she was ready for a break. Her own internal time table told her it was time for a change to a role that involved less parenting. Given Shanika's needs, however, this was not possible.

HOW PROFESSIONALS CAN HELP FAMILIES WITH HANDICAPPED CHILDREN

The overall goal of psychosocial intervention with families is to "shore up their familial strengths so that they are able to cope with the pressures placed on them by the child's handicap" (O'Hara and Levy, 1984). There are several general issues that professionals must consider to best help families in their process of adjustment.

The nature and severity of the handicap must be considered in relation to the particular family and its goals and expectations. The timing of the incident that caused the condition is crucial. Families adjusting to the birth of a handicapped child will respond somewhat differently from a family whose child was injured at a later age. In addition, the latter family may have to contend with the injured child's own response to his or her new condition. The cause of the condition is important because parents will cope differently if they think that they caused the handicapping condition. As O'Hara and Levy (1984, p. 73) point out, understanding how parents interpret the meaning of their situation is very important: "Of major importance to anyone working with the child or his parents is understanding how the family defines the situation they find themselves in. That is, how do they perceive and understand what is happening to them? It is a critical first step in planning intervention to know the degree of congruence between parents on the meaning of this child for them and the extent of the parents' uncertainty about his problems."

Parents generally need to hear the diagnostic information several times before they are able to integrate it sufficiently to feel comfortable with their understanding of it. Parents should always be given ample time and have many occasions to ask questions and express concerns and fears.

Individual members and families may benefit from individual or family counseling, psychotherapy, or group experiences. Initially, most parents are able to talk privately with a counselor or in the presence of a spouse. Group experiences are more beneficial after the initial period of adjustment to the handicapping condition. Then parents or siblings are better able to listen and benefit from the experiences of others in similar circumstances. Ultimately, a group provides realistic feedback as well as emotional nurturance to its members, and people feel a sense of increased self-esteem as they are able to help others. They learn that their feelings and behaviors are normal.

Sometimes, even very shortly after diagnosis, one or both parents may be helped by speaking with another parent or couple who are somewhat farther along in the adjustment process. This will not work for everyone, and the couple chosen to help should be very stable in their adjustment and insightful and articulate about the process they have experienced.

Couples counseling, with an educational focus, or treatment taking a more insight-oriented approach, should be considered when parents seem to be at odds over how to manage the child or if they appear to be isolated from one another. Individual treatment may be necessary, particularly if a parent seems stuck in the process or if the parental response is preventing necessary treatment for the child.

Workshops, planned by parents and professionals together, are an effective means of meeting the needs of families with handicapped children. Control is given to parents by addressing their needs as they see them, and support is provided for all family members in a way that normalizes the adjustment process.

Social case work services must be provided throughout the life cycle of the child. Initially, the social worker must play a major role in obtaining services for the handicapped child. As parents gain experience with the service delivery system, they will become more proficient in obtaining services on their own. The social worker's role then becomes one of informing parents of the existence of programs, helping them take advantage of resources, and serving as an advocate when necessary. Throughout the course of the child's life, a family will experience periods of tension, and the social worker may resume the initial role temporarily.

SUMMARY

During pregnancy, all parents entertain dreams and fantasies about their children, about how they will look and act, and about their future. Rarely do parents know before birth that their child will not be normal. When the child is born, they are unprepared for the delivery of a baby who is other than normal. The range of parental response is wide and includes shock, anger, denial, guilt, and sadness.

Most parents do adapt to the shock of having a handicapped child and do cope with the burden of care required by these children. The periods of difficulty encountered by families are largely predictable and occur at times when normal and culturally sanctioned events are taking place for others but not for their handicapped child.

The concept of the life cycle is useful because it identifies normal tasks and needs at a particular time, thereby distinguishing normal periods of stress in families from tension created or exacerbated by the presence of a handicapped child. When the problem can be identified as a normal (rather than pathological) response to a stressful life circumstance, it is possible to intervene without judgment and support a family in their ongoing adjustment to a chronic condition. Social workers and other health professionals must assume roles that meet the needs of families during the various phases of the life cycle.

REFERENCES

Bell, R.Q., and Harper, L.V. (1977). *Child effects on adults*. Hillsdale, New Jersey: Erlbaum.

Bentovim, A. (1972). Emotional disturbance of handicapped preschool children and their families: Attitudes to the child. *British Medical Journal, 3,* 579–581.

Chess, S., Fernandez, P., and Korn, S. (1980). The handicapped child and his family: Consonance and dissonance. *Journal of the American Academy of Child Psychiatry, 19,* 56–67.

Erikson, E.H. (1963). *Childhood and society* (2nd Ed.). New York: Norton.

Faerstein, L.M. (1981). Stress and coping in families of learning disabled children: A literature review. *Journal of Learning Disabilities, 14,* 420–423.

Fewell, R.R., and Gelb, S.A. (1983). Parenting moderately handicapped persons. In M. Seligman (Ed.), *The family with a handicapped child: Understanding and treatment* (pp. 175–203). New York: Grune and Stratton.

Goffman, E. (1963). *Stigma: Notes on the management of spoiled identity.* New York: Jason Aronson, Inc.

Kubler-Ross, E. (1969). *On death and dying.* New York: Macmillan.

Levine, R.A. (1980). A cross cultural perspective on parenting. In M.D. Fantini and R. Cardenas (Eds.), *Parenting in a multicultural society* (pp. 132–149). New York: Longman.

McCollum, A.T. (1984). Grieving over the lost dream. *Exceptional Parent, 14,* 9–12.

O'Hara, D.M., and Levy, J.M. (1984). Family adaptation to learning disability: A framework for understanding and treatment. *Learning Disabilities, 3,* 63–76.

Olshansky, S. (1962). Chronic sorrow: A response to having an mentally defective child. *Social Casework, 43,* 190–193.

Powell, T.H., and Ogle, P.A. (1985). *Brothers and sisters: A special part of exceptional families.* Baltimore: Brookes.

Rhodes, S.L. (1977). A developmental approach to the life cycle of the family. *Social Casework, 58,* 301–304.

Roskies, E. (1972). *Abnormality and normality: The mothering of thalidomide children.* Ithaca, New York: Cornell University Press.

Solnit, A.J., and Stark, M.H. (1961). Mourning the birth of a defective child. *Psychoanalytic Study of the Child, 16,* 523–537.

Stein, R.E.K., and Jessup, D.J. (1982). A non-categorical approach to chronic childhood illness. *Public Health Reports, 97,* 354–362.

Strickler, E. (1969). Family interaction factors in psychogenic learning disturbance. *Journal of Learning Disabilities, 2,* 31–38.

Wetter, J. (1972). Parent attitudes toward learning disability. *Exceptional Children, 38,* 490–491.

Wikler, L., Wasow, M., and Hatfield, E. (1980). Chronic sorrow revisited: Parent vs. professional depiction of the adjustment of parents of mentally retarded children. *American Journal of Orthopsychiatry, 51,* 63–70.

Willner, S.K., and Crane, R. (1979). A parental dilemma: The child with a marginal handicap. *Social Casework, 60,* 30–35.

Wolfensberger, W. (1967). Counseling the parents of the retarded. In A.A. Baumeister (Ed.), *Mental retardation: Appraisal, education and rehabilitation* (pp. 475–493). Chicago: Aldine.

INDEX